Food and Mental Health

Written by an experienced psychotherapist, this book provides professionals in the fields of health and wellbeing with a guide to human relationships with food and their impact on mental health.

Acknowledging how food choices profoundly affect a person's experience in the world, Gerrie Hughes offers knowledge and support around how to understand and negotiate the relationship between food and mind. Chapters offer facts, information and theories on key topics such as self-image, 'good' nutrition, sustainability and rituals. Each chapter uses vignettes, case studies and reflective activities to stimulate thought about the reader's own assumptions and experience and offer approaches to how they might use their expertise with the people with whom they work.

Providing an accessible and easy-to-read guide into the role food plays in our lives, this book will be of interest to a range of healthcare practitioners, including mental health nurses, occupational therapists, psychotherapists and counsellors.

Gerrie Hughes is a UKCP Registered Gestalt psychotherapist and supervisor, working in private practice since 1992. She has wide experience working in the NHS, education and business as a therapist, supervisor and facilitator.

With illustrations by Liz Hammond.

Liz Hammond trained as an existential psychoanalytic psychotherapist, working within and outside the NHS, and taught at Surrey University. She began taking lessons at the emilyball@seawhites contemporary art school about 20 years ago, has her own studio and has exhibited locally in Sussex, in London and in Wales.

Food and Mental Health
A Guide for Health Professionals

Gerrie Hughes

With illustrations by **Liz Hammond**

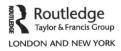

Routledge
Taylor & Francis Group

LONDON AND NEW YORK

Cover image credit:
© Liz Hammond

First published 2022
by Routledge
2 Park Square, Milton Park, Abingdon, Oxon OX14 4RN

and by Routledge
605 Third Avenue, New York, NY 10158

Routledge is an imprint of the Taylor & Francis Group, an informa business

British Library Cataloguing-in-Publication Data
A catalogue record for this book is available from the British Library

Library of Congress Cataloging-in-Publication Data
A catalog record for this book has been requested

ISBN: 978-0-367-77632-9 (hbk)
ISBN: 978-0-367-77631-2 (pbk)
ISBN: 978-1-003-17216-1 (ebk)

DOI: 10.4324/9781003172161

Typeset in Times New Roman
by Apex CoVantage, LLC

For all the grandchildren. Especially:
Arthur Mabey
Ellery Tucker
Emilia Cavazza Poli
Charlie Illes
Harry, Archie and Bella Hall
Evie and George Page

Contents

Acknowledgements   viii

Introduction   1

1   Appetizer: a taste of what is coming next   3

2   What makes 'good' nutrition: food groups and
    traditional cuisines   16

3   Roots: factors underlying relationships with food   29

4   Wholeness, balance and regulation: needs and Gestalt   50

5   A world of food: history and current situation   74

6   Difference and diversity   93

7   Vital and virtual: personal and digital relationships   119

8   Rituals and feasts: food, art and spirituality   141

9   Digestif: satisfaction and integration   157

Index   169

Acknowledgements

Thanks to those who have contributed their own experiences.

Rachel David

Di Hodgson

Mary Hughes

Piergiulio Poli

Jo Shah

Sharon Usher

Kevin Williamson

Amanda Wood

Photographer: Bill Phillip

Introduction

If you are reading this, you probably know that food is significant for mental health. You may be surprised, as I was, by quite how significant it is. You may also be thinking that you lack information and skills around the topic that might make you a more effective practitioner. This would not be surprising. It is only now that the medical profession is beginning to train new doctors in how to help patients eat better in order to regain physical and mental health. Alternatively, you may already have a great deal of expertise in the fields of diet and nutrition, in which case, the book may offer a different perspective that could be refreshing.

Certainly, in my own experience of training as a Gestalt psychotherapist, we talked about food a lot as a metaphor for how we engage with life generally, but there was no training in how the lack of certain nutrients in a diet can be an underlying cause of depression and anxiety and other mental health conditions that bring people into therapy on an everyday basis. My approach to practice has changed as I have been learning about brain chemistry and soil quality.

Food is a delight, and it is also a challenge. I don't know how many times, when I told people I was writing a book about food and mental health, they looked guilty and turned away, as if I was judging their size and weight. This is not a book about judgement and certainly not about critiquing how health professionals set about their work. Instead, it is an overview of the context in which we practise: an exploration of mental health and what it means for us as individuals and as a society, using food as the focal reference.

This is meant as a practical book: experience near, moment by moment, everyday explorations of the interactions practitioners have with a whole range of patients, clients and service users: how difference (and sameness) may influence the contact, and some observations about how and, maybe, why this can happen. It will explore the various facets of mental health, bringing together the ingredients needed for a satisfying life.

Many of the factors that influence health and wellbeing are environmental ones. Not only the natural environment, but also the social and regulatory environment, which has such an influence on those who have access to food and those who do not, or who have only limited access.

It can be the case that health professionals know and understand many models of ill-health and how to treat it. In this book, I present a model of what good health

DOI: 10.4324/9781003172161-1

may look like in a human being. Not far into writing it, I realized that physical and mental health are the same thing in many respects. Building mental and emotional resilience can help us deal with any acute or chronic physical illnesses and conditions that may befall us. Taking care of the body with good nutrition and appropriate exercise can also support us through conditions that affect our mental health.

The book is also a glimpse into someone else's relationship with food as I share the small, everyday, food-related rituals that bring me meaning and satisfaction. I describe my struggles and successes in the attempt to achieve a life that is simple, graceful and regulated.

1 Appetizer

A taste of what is coming next

Introduction

The words we use about food are the same ones we use about life: abundance, hunger, appetite, taste, disgust, satisfaction and more. Food is, literally, essential for life, but our relationships with it, both individually and collectively, can become problematic. When they do, the result is disease, distress and strain on services. We are accustomed to making the link between what and how we eat and our physical health but, currently, researchers are recognizing the link between food and mental health.

Thinking about it, this seems obvious – we are whole people, not just the sum of our parts. We are also fundamentally interconnected with our environments. Eating (along with breathing) is one of the basic ways that this relatedness is experienced. Sometimes I think this deep interdependence is difficult to perceive, like when an object is so close to your face it can't be seen properly. This lack of clarity means we go along with ideas that, if we could let ourselves accept the reality of them, would dismay us.

As individuals, we make food choices that we know, at some level, do not really nourish our bodies. Like when I slather butter on pieces of white bread (albeit home-made organic sourdough) to make a sandwich for lunch because I'm hungry, tired and having to process everything that happened with my work that morning. I have beautiful organic lettuce in my fridge, and the wherewithal to make a healthy salad. But what I'm hungry for at that moment is comfort, and my body remembers my grandmother giving me butter on everything. Our bodies and minds need nourishment on many different levels and, I suppose, there is something helpful for me in at least being able to bring my choices into awareness, even if I still make the 'bad' ones.

This dissonance also happens for us as a society. In Britain, we seem to have arrived at a position where what food needs most to be is cheap. Never mind if it means that people or animals are exploited to produce it, or if potentially harmful fertilizers or pesticides are involved, or if it only tastes reasonable because it contains a lot of sugar or salt, so long as it is at the lowest price compared with competitors. I understand that the beneficial intention behind this approach is to

DOI: 10.4324/9781003172161-2

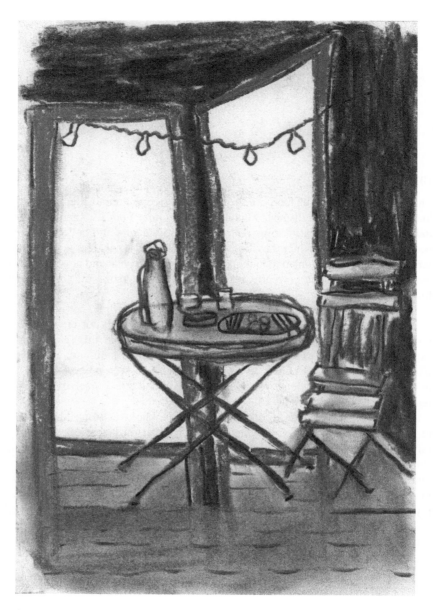

Setting out the table

avoid those on low incomes having to go hungry, but then I wonder about what it takes for people to be truly nourished.

What can we do?

This book is offered as a guide for professionals whose role is to facilitate others to understand their relationship with the world and to support them in making that relationship as satisfying as possible – which means, from my point of view, satisfying for both individual and world. I don't think just satisfying one side of the relationship is sustainable anymore. You may be a therapist, doctor, nurse, teacher, sports coach or a parent wanting to help your family build satisfying relationships with food for the future (remembering, though, that this book focuses on working with adults). You may have noticed that your patients, clients, students or family are involved in challenging negotiations with their diet and their physical and mental health. In this work, I'm attempting to identify and describe areas of experience that may be relevant for us all, whichever side of the 'helping' relationship we are on at a particular time. To this exploration, you will, I hope, feel able to bring your own experience, expertise and preferences. For ease of expression, from now on I will talk about 'professionals', hoping to encompass all the disciplines that this kind of material would interest, and 'client', which means anyone to whom we have a contractual commitment or responsibility.

Why I wrote the book

There is something daring about offering a book to a multi-disciplinary readership. Inevitably, there is a risk that readers will have far greater expertise than I do in neuroscience, physiology, nutrition and many other fields. The expertise I do claim for myself comes from having worked with people for 30 years as a Gestalt psychotherapist, with the aim of making lives that are more satisfying for all of us. Counsellors and psychotherapists may not know everything about how to provide effective support in every context but being and working in relationship with others is the discipline we practise; it is where our training and professional development is focused and what our accrediting organizations assess.

When I wrote my previous book, 'Competence and Self-care in Counselling and Psychotherapy', which was published by Routledge in 2014, it was designed directly for my own profession. Yet, when I had finished it, I realized it could be useful to anyone who works with others: managers, teachers, social workers, HR and sales professionals, for example. Most jobs require that people work with others, whether as leaders, facilitators, or colleagues or with customers. My focus in that book turned out to be too narrow and it feels important to focus on a wider readership this time. Besides, it seems to me that the traditional boundaries between disciplines and, indeed, art and science are no longer relevant or practical and that people must be versatile and open to learning across subject boundaries throughout their lifetimes.

If you had told me ten years ago that I would be researching and writing about the brain, I would have been horrified. Yet, when the neuroscientists started discovering the link between mirror neurons and empathy, I felt like science was 'proving' something I already knew as a therapist. A similar thing happened when I started to read about the work of scientists linking mental health and diet. The findings were in tune with my subjective experience as a person who eats, who shops and cooks for myself and my friends and family, and who also works with others around their relationship with food.

Difficulties and delights around food have been a major issue in my own life. They have also figured very largely in my work with clients. This seems like the right time to bring together what I have learned.

Words and meaning

Before going any further, I would like to clarify something about the terms I use and what underlies my approach. To begin with, some terms. You may not define these words in the same way because of your own professional training or personal preference, and I don't think that matters particularly. But it seems important to me to be clear about what I mean when I use them.

- **Brain.** This is the organ that dwells in our skulls – the physical, cellular matter.
- **Gut.** Following the outcomes of research in the late twentieth century, deeper understanding of the significance of microorganisms present in the gut and the connection between brain and gut via the vagus nerve, has led to new thinking about how human beings operate internally and also how we engage with our environments. The gut microbiome is a garden of organisms that are not us, but that co-exist intimately within our digestive tracts to help us assimilate what we take in (and not only food) (Mayer, 2016).
- **Mind.** The subjective experience of the operation of the brain and gut **plus**, for me, the experience of the body, a lot of which, like the movement of blood, is out of awareness. The physical body is in constant exchange with the environment, breathing and sensing, held by gravity. Tim Parks expresses this beautifully in his book 'Out of my Head' (Parks, 2018), in which he describes his journeys as a layperson into some of the current scientific beliefs about the brain and consciousness. For him, 'mind is the happening of body and environment together' (p. 33).
- **Psychological.** Matters concerned with my rational, cognitive experience of being. Some definitions (including the one I just looked up on Wikipedia) include emotional experience in them. While I know we are whole beings, and that to attempt to dismantle us into constituent parts diminishes our nature, for the purposes of this exploration I would like to be able to differentiate the mental and emotional aspects of our engagement with the world so as to understand them better.
- **Emotional.** My embodied, intuitive experience of being, where rationality is irrelevant.

- **Senses.** The conduits through which I experience being in the world. These are, of course, sight, hearing, touch, taste, smell, plus the proprioceptive sense of what I am experiencing in my body.
- **Self.** My experience of body and mind interrelating with other beings and the world over time, and in this present time and place. By this, I mean the personal history that has made me what I am today, plus how the person I am now influences the possibilities available to me in the current moment and, importantly, the potential I have to learn, grow and change for the future.

Food and mental health

There is a range of areas of human experience around which food and our brains, bodies and minds are connected. Here is a brief overview of the areas I will be exploring in the following chapters.

Food and the brain

Sloshing around the brain is a cerebral fluid, composed of water and fats, that protects the precious structures, delivers nutrients and washes away waste. The brain needs food in order to keep working and glucose is its only form of sustenance. In fact, the brain takes 20% of the body's glucose supplies, although it is only 2% of its weight (Carter, 2019). This glucose comes from the food we eat that contains sugar and starch, found in fruit, vegetables and grains. These carbohydrates can be divided into two types, simple and complex. Simple carbohydrates, refined sugar, for example, are quickly processed by the digestive system and provide an immediate burst of energy, but the available energy soon drops, and the body begins to crave for another sugar hit. In contrast, complex carbs, like potatoes and other vegetables, fruit, brown rice and grains, are more steadily processed by the body and so provide a more sustained form of energy. People often call this difference in processing 'GI' (glycaemic index). The fast processors are high GI and the slow are low. Consistent, steady supplies of energy are important for the body, but for the brain, they are essential. **The brain reacts to lack of glucose in the same way that it reacts to lack of oxygen** (Carter, 2019).

The processing cells of the brain are called neurons. They resemble straggly stars with branched points. One of the points is longer and thicker than the others, reaching out into a web of connection with other neurons. This is an axion. Along the axion, there are points called synapses, small gaps between the neurons which are the areas of communication between them. One of the ways they communicate is by chemicals called neurotransmitters. There are many different types of neurotransmitters that tend to excite or inhibit (send or block) nerve impulses. Familiar examples include serotonin, dopamine and noradrenaline (Carter, 2019). **The raw materials to manufacture neurotransmitters come from the food we eat.**

Serotonin is a neurotransmitter that is connected with mood, appetite and sleep and so is important for general wellbeing. It is produced from tryptophan, an amino acid that is found in protein sources of food like meat, fish and grains (more about food groups will be found in Chapter 2). However, in order to cross the blood-brain barrier, which protects the brain from any toxins that might be circulating in the blood, the presence of carbohydrate (from vegetables, grains, etc.) is necessary. Once across the barrier, folic acid, vitamin B_6, biotin (another kind of B vitamin) and zinc are all essential for the final transformation into serotonin (Geary, 2001). Folic acid comes from vegetables and the other nutrients come from meat and eggs (Leyse-Wallace, 2008).

Depression, anxiety, schizophrenia, autism, Alzheimer's disease and Parkinson's disease have all been connected with dietary deficiencies. Scientists are currently conducting research programmes that build a solid evidence base for identifying nutrients that benefit the brain and substances that are detrimental. For example, Professor Felice Jacka, a groundbreaking researcher in the field (https://foodandmoodcentre.com.au), offers a thorough and accessible overview of the current international situation in her book 'Brainchanger' (2019, Yellow Kite).

Food and the gut

It's breakfast time and I've just eaten a bowl of porridge with walnuts and maple syrup. I can see the empty bowl on the table beside me. The transformation of that bowl of creamy grains and gnarly nuts into glucose to feed my brain and provide energy for the activities I need to perform is one of those everyday miracles that it is easy to take for granted. Allowing something 'foreign' into the complex conglomeration of matter and energy that I recognize as being 'me' is potentially fraught with risk. Who knows what harmful substances may lurk there unnoticed? This is where the microorganisms that live in my gut come into their own. The spoonful of porridge studded with little walnut shards that I put in my mouth mixes with saliva and receives some attention from my teeth before it slides into my stomach and then onwards through my intestinal tract. The microorganisms lining the whole route recognize toxins and deal with them; they also work out exactly how to process all the other nourishing substances I have ingested, as well as checking out how things are going generally with the whole organism by means of a two-way communication with the brain. The quality of my emotional state is taken into account. This morning I was relaxed and able to give the process of eating a lot of my attention (alongside wondering casually what exactly I might write as I tackled this section). Another morning, I might gulp down my porridge as quickly as possible before attending to an urgent demand to deal with something else. In those circumstances, the feelings of warm satisfaction I am currently experiencing around my middle may instead be sensations of lumpy acidity. . . . Incidentally, the largest supplies of the neurotransmitter serotonin, the regulator of appetite, mood and sleep, are found in the gut and not in the brain (Mayer, 2016).

I inherited my microbiome from my mother, from the birth canal when I was born; thus, although I can't possibly know whether any of the descendants of her microorganisms are actually still present, my body has the potential to carry generational information in my gut, as well as in my DNA. Babies born by caesarean lose out on that direct transmission, therefore they have to create microbiota for themselves from their environments (Mayer, 2016). I imagine the microbiome to be a bit like the sourdough culture I keep in my fridge, ready for when I want to make bread. The 'mother-leaven' ('madre-lievito' is the word Italians use) bread culture was originally given to me by David at the local bakery, who handed it over in an old yoghurt container. I began to feed it with my own choice of flour and, over time, it has incorporated other microorganisms from my skin, and from my kitchen, transforming it into something uniquely connected to me and my environment (Kimbell, 2017). This means bread made from it is particularly wholesome and digestible for me and family. Antibiotics decimate the microbiome. Foods that help cultivate it are the fermented ones like kefir and sauerkraut.

Inflammation is a bodily response that highlights important considerations for our understanding of the impact of our western lifestyles. In some ways, I think of it as being like the stress response, which is our bodies' way of reacting to the danger of being attacked from outside. It is probably widely understood now that the nature of our lifestyles can mean that our stress response is constantly 'on', rather than switching off when the danger has past, which goes against the way our bodies have evolved and so can eventually become harmful to us. Inflammation is how we respond both to threats from outside that have actually made it inside and to threats coming from inside. It involves the release of protein substances called cytokines, which regulate the response of the immune system to the intrusion. Gut microbes have a big part to play in this process. They examine every item of food we ingest for harmful substances and alert the immune system to be ready to deal with them. They also work with the immune system to neutralize other sources of harmful bacteria coming into the body, from a cut finger, for example. When injury happens on the outside of our bodies, like the cut finger, we can see the redness and swelling which is the immune system's way of dealing with the situation. We need this to keep us alive but, like the stress response, our diets can mean that inflammation never switches 'off', so it becomes chronic. Acute inflammation, like the flow of adrenalin triggered by the nervous system to make us ready to counter external threats, is healthy. Chronic inflammation, like a chronic stress response, can cause physical and mental ill-health. Stress levels are known to heighten inflammation, and inflammation is connected with depression.

The foods that trigger inflammation are refined sugar and grains, alcohol, caffeine and processed foods generally. Substances called probiotics are believed to help with soothing inflammation. These are the 'live' parts of yoghurt and are also available as supplements (Ash, 2014). Further information is available on the National Health Service (NHS) website on probiotics. I return to the involvement microorganisms have in our lives in Chapter 5. A more detailed (and very accessible) explanation of the gut microbiome, inflammation and the immune system can be found in 'The Hidden Half of Nature' by David R. Montgomery and Anne Biklé (published by Norton in 2016).

Thinking about food

Food nutrients are crucial for the continued smooth running of our brains, as well as the rest of our bodies. But where do the nutrients in the foods themselves come from? From the soil we grow our food in. Intensive farming methods mean that nutrients taken from the soil are not replaced (more in Chapter 5). This means that the vegetables we eat directly, and the animals we eat that are themselves fed on depleted food, cannot provide us with the essentials for a healthy life.

Our society's relationship with food seems to have become disordered. What we eat is already affecting our physical and mental wellbeing. There is so much in the media these days about overweight and obesity, and other 'lifestyle' conditions. The solutions being offered seem to involve regulating the food industry to influence a change in that outcome. The UK government's approach to resolving this disconnect between what is available for us to eat and what we need to become healthy as a society can be found on the National Food Strategy's website.

We also hear about the prevalence of eating disorders, particularly among young people (see more information on the anorexiabulimiacare website). They are so prevalent that, as well as maybe working with clients experiencing issues, we may know people with difficulties around eating or experience them ourselves. We see images of very slim people on our screens and countless plates of meals about to be enjoyed on social media. We allow our eating choices to be influenced by all this information. Then sometimes we don't. And sometimes we can't. We are surrounded by discussions and contradictions about food, and the way we handle them can influence our general wellbeing and maybe our mental health. More about eating disorders will be found in Chapter 3.

It seems to me that something is missing in society's approach to food awareness, and those of us who facilitate others around these issues may have a contribution to make to easing the situation. Yet we know that change is difficult for us as individuals, even when we understand it's for our own benefit. (I don't think I can be the only person in the health professions to feel this way. . . .)

Facilitating/encouraging/motivating/advising/persuading/inspiring/helping other people to make changes is a whole other skill set, one that is probably fundamental to all our roles, in different ways. This book is meant as a resource for thinking about our personal and societal situation and about relationships with food and how we can work most effectively with clients in our own individual situations

Feelings about food

Are you happy about your body weight? When I ask myself that question now, the answer I come up with is sometimes. . . . It depends on the context I'm in and how I experience it. For much of my life, though, the answer would definitely have been 'no'. But I would have done anything not to ask myself that question. And if I had been asked by someone else, a doctor, for example, I would have collapsed into shame and denial and 'disappeared' from the situation emotionally. Our clients will very likely have their own individual emotional reactions to conversations about food. Sometimes these might even clash with ours, which could be a barrier to a successful outcome. Some models that may be useful for understanding interpersonal dynamics and how to use them in the service of our clients will be introduced later on in the book. Hopefully they will offer a fresh perspective on what it means to engage with another person around their (and perhaps our) vulnerabilities.

Sensing and food

All our senses are engaged around food. Ideally, a meal is a delight in every aspect: nourishing, satisfying, energizing and shared with those we love. Unfortunately, this is not always how it turns out. Yet our senses are the most accessible means we have for choosing what we eat and calibrating our intake. Re-enlivening appetite through connection with the senses can enable greater satisfaction and enjoyment, and re-build trust in our bodies' knowing.

Food and the wider environment

The use of land and farming techniques is easy to understand as being relevant to humans' relationship with food, so also are the distribution mechanisms for the arrival of products in supermarkets, smaller shops and local markets. We seem hardly to think about them and just take for granted they will happen until something occurs that draws them to our attention – like the 2020 Covid-19 pandemic. Then all our primitive fears surface and we strip supermarket shelves and hoard. We are connected to our environment: if the land that grows our food or the logistics that connect us with it are under threat, then we as human beings are under threat too.

Less obvious connections are the relationship with politics and global finance, and transport infrastructure. Yet we all know at some level that where we live affects what food is available to us. The history of the world, colonialism, natural resources and current political environments all have an impact on what arrives on our plate at meal times – if there is a plate, and if we have access to food at all.

Increased awareness and understanding of how these issues affect our daily experience may redirect the guilt and shame that seems to be present around food into appropriate, addressable concerns. I am speaking for myself here as a beneficiary of a lot of political and financial advantages.

I also explore how the prevalence of internet and social media affects both digital and face-to-face interactions. How do we and our clients reject or assimilate the limitless input from our devices?

Food, difference and diversity

While the need for food is something we share with all living beings, what we eat, and where and how, can also be a significant separator. Understanding the dynamics around meal times can be a potent way of exposing injustices, one that is available to most of us several times a day.

Food and art

From earliest times, our ancestors depicted food in their creative works. We know this because the cave paintings of the animals they hunted are still there for us to see. Whether fruit, vegetables and meat are depicted as a representation of themselves, or as a symbol conveying a hidden meaning, foodstuffs have long been objects of interest to visual artists.

Then there is food as art. As well as the design of a recipe, the execution of a dish and the arrangement of a plate, there is the artistry of writing about food. Television programmes about cooking and celebrity chefs are part of the culture now. Fine art, culinary arts and the literature around food, whether it is a recipe, a magazine article or a description of a meal eaten by a character in a novel, all contribute to our experience of being, shape who we are as individuals and also influence our shared culture.

Food and spirituality

My family were immigrants into South Wales from Ireland, and I was brought up as a Roman Catholic. Our most important celebration of worship, the mass, was designed around a meal – the last supper of Jesus Christ, on the evening before his crucifixion, when he consecrated bread and wine and called them his own body and blood. As a child, I also remember witnessing the sacred Friday meal at the home of my Jewish friend. I was allowed to wait while the family lit candles, prayed and ate what was for me highly exotic food, so that Linda and I could begin playing together again immediately after they had finished. I have also witnessed the tense faces of Muslim friends and colleagues during Ramadan and followed a path of little lights into dinner at Diwali. Then there are the secular rituals of family suppers, Christmas dinners and birthday teas, the symbology of table, candles and the shopping basket.

Structure for the book

Approach to practice

While researching for this book, I came to understand how food is intrinsic to every part of life: religion, history, finance, politics, the arts, race, class, the landscape, power and much more. Inevitably, when exploring an area of such breadth, the different constituent elements become the focus for a time. Yet we are whole beings, interconnected with our environment, and the choices we make at one level have consequences for the rest, whether that concerns our bodies' internal mechanisms or our relationships with other people and the wider world.

When we meet our clients, we are both interacting with them in the present moment and intervening in their wider life situation. As a therapist, I look for feedback from my clients about how their experience of the world 'out there' is changing during the time we are meeting together for sessions.

These interrelationships are complex and make the idea of cause and effect irrelevant. While I was writing my previous book, I arrived at a framework for understanding what effectiveness may look like when working with other people in complex, dynamic situations (like life). It was a threefold model of practitioner (professional), client and context. Each of these elements contributes to a satisfying outcome, although what seems to work well depends largely on context. I guess most health professionals would recognize that responses that work wonderfully well in some situations are disastrous in others. Taking all three elements into account in professional decision making helps us to respond appropriately to the here-and-now situation. While working with our clients, we make choices all the time: for example, about what to say and how to express it, conceptualizing the issues involved in the situation they are bringing to us to relieve, and applying skilfully what we know in order to help alleviate the difficulty. A lot of this happens out of awareness, in the heat of the moment.

We can bring it into awareness through reflective practice. The exciting thing for me about reflective practice is that by doing it, I can understand the new learning I have gained from my day-to-day work activities (Bager-Charlson, 2012). This is important because it is how advances in skills and knowledge are recognized by individual practitioners and current significant themes for the professions are identified. This book is an invitation into reflective practice around food and mental health

Each chapter will focus on one, or some, of these aspects. It will gather together information that I believe you will find relevant for your client group or for yourself. At the end of each chapter, some personal experience around the topic will be shared. There will also be suggestions for activities that you can participate in personally and/or offer to your clients. The chapter will close with a food note – maybe a connection with the food I am cooking and eating while writing this book, or a recipe for a dish that is mentioned somewhere in the text, so you have the opportunity to taste it for yourself, if that appeals to you.

Chapter summary

Food is a powerful connector between individuals and the world. While exploring that relationship, insight may be gained into the person's general relationship with every facet of their lives. It may also highlight society's structures and assumptions, offering a vivid reflection of the culture in general. Our mental health is influenced by both our personal experience and the society in which we are embedded.

Professionals will be invited to reflect on their own experience by means of information and ideas around a range of areas of exploration. Some specific activities or exercises will be offered as a means of further examination and some personal reflections will be included as possible examples. Finally, a short section will be devoted just to the enjoyment of food.

The ingredients and method presented here will be about how to make a satisfying life, rather than an enjoyable meal, although each is so dependent on the other as to be inseparable.

Activities

Please consider the following questions. This may involve thinking about them, meditating on them or making a piece of free-flowing, uncensored writing, similar to those in a personal journal.

1.1 How would I describe my relationship to food and eating?

1.2 What do I want to be the outcome of my work with clients?

1.3 Try to distil your response to question 1.2 into one short phrase or sentence. You may want to share this with me and other readers on social media, as a way of participating in a conversation. Maybe find a food item, a piece of kitchen equipment or a favourite meal that illustrates your approach and post it and your distilled response on Instagram using the hashtag #foodandmentalhealth.

1.4 How does my profession use reflective practice?

Personal reflection

It has taken me a long time to gather the ingredients for this book. Years ago, I read the stories of writers who went to Italy to eat and cook, and then I went to Italy to eat and cook several times myself, although not always to the same places. I had a deep desire to learn how to write like a food-writer. For me, this meant conveying in words the deep experience of the senses: the charm of conviviality and the sturdiness of the kitchen table. I think that could be a life's work – as understanding the effect on our minds and bodies of what and how we eat is.

My relationship with food had already been long and fraught. I was a fat child when everyone else was thin. I was searingly sensitive to too much, or too little, but powerless to change my relationship with food. This had an effect on my relationship with people too. I believed that my acceptance by others was profoundly conditional: many people told me I would be really pretty if I wasn't so fat. I knew I was vulnerable to disdain because I was called names all the time, 'tubs', 'fatty', 'fatso' . . . Buying school uniform was an ordeal because I was too big for the regular sizes. One afternoon, walking home from primary school with a group of classmates, I was targeted by one of the boys who started calling me names, and then punching me, as hard as he could in what we both probably considered to be my offensively fat stomach. I might have just walked off and joined the others, but I didn't.

I only managed to lose my excess weight when my parents had both died, which is a curious thing for me – I don't understand it rationally, yet it is poignantly meaningful. Then I began my journeys to Italy and other places, and I could enjoy the food, and admit to it with a clear conscience at last, even to write about it. I believe food can and should be one of life's great joys, but I know it can be complicated.

Food note

'Whole' food

As I begin to write this book, I've noticed that I prefer now to use whole garlic cloves and even whole red chillies in the food I cook. My style of cooking is usually to start by chopping an onion, 'melting' it in olive oil in a pan (by this I mean cooking it slowly so that the fragments become transparent and meld together) and spreading a little salt over the food to release the juices, as I was taught by Carla Tomasi in Rome. Then I sling in some chickpeas, brown lentils or whatever pulses I have in the fridge, some spices and some oil or liquid to cook. I used to chop garlic and chillies, but putting them in whole and cooking everything slowly, particularly in the presence of a good oil, makes the softened cloves burst pungently and the chillies collapse off their stalks with a flash of heat. Whole is good.

References

Ash, M. (2014) 'Resolving depression: The role of the gut in taming inflammation', in Watts, M. (ed.) *Nutrition and mental health: A handbook*. Hove: Pavilion.

Bager-Charlson, S. (2012) *Personal development in counselling and psychotherapy*. London: Sage.

Carter, R. (2019) *The brain book*. London: Dorling Kindersley.

Geary, A. (2001) *The food and mood handbook*. London: Thorsons.

Jacka, F. (2019) *Brainchanger*. Great Britain: Yellow Kite.

Kimbell, V. (2017) *The sourdough school*. London: Kyle Books.

Leyse-Wallace, R. (2008) *Linking nutrition to mental health*. Lincoln, NE: iUniverse.

Mayer, E. (2016) *The mind-gut connection*. New York: Harper Collins.

Montgomery, D.R. and Biklé, A. (2016) *The hidden half of nature*. London: Norton & Co.

Parks, T. (2018) *Out of my head*. London: Harvill Secker.

2 What makes 'good' nutrition

Food groups and traditional
cuisines

Introduction

Satisfaction is many-levelled, nuanced and provisional. Put another way, the kind of nourishment that suits a person in one particular place and moment can become distasteful or even disgusting in another. This is appropriate, essential even, because it is part of the way we regulate our choices, enabling ourselves to provide our bodies and minds with what is necessary for growth, wellbeing and a satisfying life. While there probably never has been a perfect world in which it was possible to regulate food intake impeccably, present-day western society – the way we live now – makes balance and therefore satisfaction challenging. Food is easily available and, often, the kind of food that is available is tempting but not necessarily best for our bodies, leaving us with a dilemma. Do I feed my hunger by the instantly satisfying bite of an almond croissant, or do I feed the satisfaction I experience from comfortable digestion, a feeling of lightness and maintaining my weight at a reasonable level? These are choices I face several times each day. (I sometimes cut the almond croissant in half and share it with a friend, or else keep the bit I don't eat in the freezer for another time, when I just feel the need for something sweet and flaky again. . . .) Of course, in other parts of the world food is not so easily available and people face different challenges.

Whatever our food environment, our appetites and pleasure are our personal, internal guides to what we want and need to eat – influenced by what is available. Being informed about the likely consequences of our choices can help us make them more satisfying, and the kind of knowledge that we are likely to need is an understanding of food groups and the nature of the nutrition that each provides. Then there is the energy we take from what we eat, usually talked about in terms of calories; generally, the more active we are, the greater the amount of calories we need to consume, although I've noticed that I sometimes need to eat more, and different things, when I'm recovering from illness or injury. Most of us are aware of food groups and calorie content, but it is sometimes useful to revisit what we think we know in a different context.

The focus of this book is on facilitating others around issues of food and mental health, so it seems important to consider the nutritional type and amount of food we eat in a way that recognizes the impact of relationships with others (including,

DOI: 10.4324/9781003172161-3

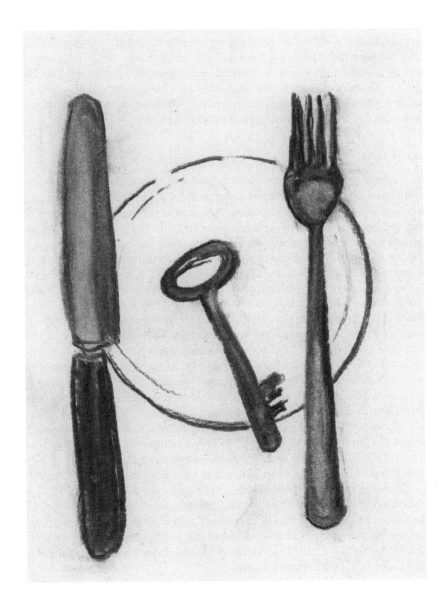

Bringing in the meal

and especially, the relationship in the room between practitioner and client) and the wider environment in which food production and consumption takes place. This approach reflects the three elements of the competence framework, introduced in Chapter 1, which are practitioner, client and context. Consequently, the chapter begins with considering food categories and energy values in context and holistically, highlighting how the shared experience of practitioner and client might be similar or different. The discussion then moves on to cuisines like the Mediterranean diet and towards understanding the lifestyle that supports it and other traditional ways of producing and consuming food.

Food groups

What we eat is usually categorized into the major groups of protein, carbohydrate, fats, fibre and vitamins and minerals. One mouthful of food usually contains a mix of some or all of those, so I want to talk about nutrition in a slightly different way. Separating anything into categories in order to understand it better is a helpful approach, but it can sometimes be useful to consider the context and bigger picture too. As I discuss the different food groups in the following sections, I describe their main effects on the human body, how we in the UK might access the foods associated with them and, where appropriate, explain how their production affects the parts of the world, or people, associated with it.

There is something, too, about the psychological and emotional impact of the choices we make and whether they are in accordance with our ethics and values system. The production of food at industrialized levels has consequences for the environment. Anything that upsets the ecology of our world has eventually to have an effect on us as individuals, however indirectly. It is easy for any of us, and I include myself in this, to feel compromised when we think about the actions society takes in our name. Then sometimes, it becomes so problematic that the only possible solution is to stop thinking about it, but this has consequences too. I explore the implications of intensive food production and develop some of the themes introduced here later on in the book (see Chapter 5).

If you are looking for a more specific and scientific discussion of how the different food groups relate to mental health, then Ruth Leyse-Wallace's (2008) 'Linking Nutrition to Mental Health' offers this, together with a history of research into the topic and an overview of specific relevant publications. If you are looking for more specific corelations between individual nutrients and the foods in which they are found, Leslie Korn's (2016) 'Nutrition Essentials for Mental Health' has useful tables for looking up specific items.

Water

Whether it is consumed as a cup of tea, a sip of water from a bottle, even a fizzy drink from a can, or a glass of wine with dinner, our bodies need water. Foods themselves have a water content: a bowl of porridge for breakfast is obviously 'wetter' than a slice of toast. The actual percentage of water content of our bodies has a wide range of between 45% and 75%, depending on factors like gender and age. More information can be found on the Medical News Today's website, where you can find an article entitled 'what percentage of the human body is water'. Interestingly, this study identifies that the brain is made up of 80% to 85% water. Water is also essential for the process of digestion, and we need to drink 2 litres of water a day to keep hydration at optimal level (Geary, 2001). This is actually quite a lot. When I measured my water intake (excluding tea, coffee and other drinks that cannot be taken into account because their other contents, like caffeine and sugar, have an effect on the body), I found it quite hard to drink that much. Nevertheless, I find the benefits of trying to drink more water outweigh the effort, and I try to drink hot water with lemon first thing in the morning and often sip constantly from a cup of warm water as I am writing or cooking.

The balance of water in our bodies is constantly regulated by sensations of thirst or the need to visit the bathroom. Sometimes we can ignore these signals for long periods. I've often heard people say, 'I've been so busy, I haven't had a drink or been to the loo all day'. We learn how to desensitize as very young children, of course, and the ability to do so is necessary, but it can be revealing to bring into awareness how we relate to these signals from our bodies and to the assumptions that are traditional for our cultures.

Access to drinkable water influences the way we live. Water is essential for life, so drought, pollution or misappropriation of available natural water is a serious threat to the people directly involved, to the planet and consequently to those of us not (yet) directly affected by lack of water.

Fibre

While it is generally categorized as a complex carbohydrate (Leyse-Wallace, 2008), I have chosen to discuss fibre separately because this is the ballast that moves what we eat through our digestive system and is much of what comes out the other end. It is found in plants, and we need a lot of it both for ease of digestion and for feelings of satisfaction. I remember, years ago, when I was training to be a psychotherapist, I was at a workshop with other trainees, and things were getting challenging, as they often did. It was lunchtime and most of us were eating the sandwiches we had brought. One of the participants sat down with a wide mixing-bowl full of chopped up vegetables and fruit and began chomping her way through it. We must all have looked surprised because she responded, 'I've been working on it with my therapist. When I'm stressed, I want to eat, but I don't want to put on weight, so I can feel satisfied if I eat a lot of low-calorie food. . .'. It clearly worked for her as a strategy and I often think about it when my own feelings of stress make me want to eat cake. . .

The environment in which we experience the fruit and vegetables for our table – fields and orchards, markets and greengrocers, supermarkets, or gardens, if we are lucky – depends on where and how we live. The nature of the fruits and vegetables and how they are grown may differ according to where we are in the world but it seems important for mental and physical wellbeing, and for our individual and societal relationships with food, to be able to connect the produce we eat with where and how it is grown.

Protein

Protein is essential for tissue growth and repair and healthy brain functioning. It is found mainly in meat, fish and pulses (peas, beans and lentils), although traces of it are found in potatoes and avocadoes and some other vegetables and grains too. Dairy products and eggs also contain protein, as well as fat. Protein also helps provide feelings of fullness and satisfaction after eating.

Meat

This is animal flesh. In the UK, we have traditionally eaten beef, lamb, pork and chicken, although other traditions and cultures eat different animals. Here, and in other 'developed' countries, a lot of the meat we eat is mass-produced and may contain antibiotics and other chemicals. These days, we mostly eat muscle in the form of a joint or chops. As a child, I remember regularly being given liver and kidneys to eat, and my father was very fond of tripe (stomach lining) and sweet-breads (testicles). I still love black pudding (made with blood) although I have purposely not to think about it on the odd occasion when I do eat it. Fatty cuts, like breast of lamb and pork belly, seem to be less popular these days too, prob-ably because animal fat has some risks for health, although eating gently roasted 'porchetta' in Sicily a few years ago reminded me of how delicious these cuts can be. The parts of animals humans don't want to eat (or that may be unsafe for us to eat) become sausages, pies, faggots, etc., or cat and dog food. Less common sources of meat, like rabbit or game, venison and ostrich, are being explored as potentially healthier alternatives to the traditional British diet.

Fish

Most fish has to be harvested from the wild, although salmon farming has become popular in recent years. Salmon is classed as an oily fish, along with tuna, kippers, mackerel, etc. Oily fish are an important source of omega-3 fatty acids, which are essential for brain and body health. Cod, plaice, sea-bass and other 'white fish' have their own category. There are also shellfish: oysters, crab, lobster, prawns, mussels, cockles, winkles and others. The type of fresh fish available depends on where you live. I have seen people picking cockles off the South Wales beaches at low tide and bought saucers of cooked ones from the local market to eat with vinegar and pepper. An Australian friend of mine (from New South Wales, inci-dentally) remembers prising oysters off a rock, splitting them open and swallow-ing the contents in one gelatinous, salty hit. Some people live many miles from the sea, but may have access to rivers and the opportunity to catch the fish that inhabit them locally. Unless I am at the seaside near a fishing area or familiar with the supplier, I mostly buy frozen fish. The frozen option can provide access to fish from further afield. I also sometimes enjoy tinned salmon and tuna. Salmon sandwiches and pickled onions were a particular favourite in my family of origin, and I like to revisit that tradition sometimes.

Taste and the nutritional quality of the fish are, of course, dependent on the waters in which they grow. For those of us who like to eat fish, unpolluted seas and rivers are important. Along with protein, fish has other valuable nutrients, like oils and vitamins and minerals, which will be discussed in later sections.

Pulses

These are traditionally peas, beans and lentils but protein is also found in grains (rice, quinoa, etc.), nuts and some vegetables. In the UK, we are accustomed to peas and beans being available in season. Fresh peas, still in their pods, are a treat for a few weeks in early summer, but they are available unpodded and frozen all year. Broad beans and long 'french' beans are similarly available. Sometimes, borlotti beans in their pink, marbled pods are available for a short time in specialist greengrocers. Runner beans winding up their wooden stakes are still a common sight in gardens and allotments providing abundant late summer harvests of food to swap and share.

I have never seen a chickpea in a pod. In this country, they usually come dried in packs and need to be soaked and boiled before being eaten, or else ready cooked in cans or jars. Many other beans are available in this way: red kidney, borlotti, cannellini, black-eyed, pinto, haricot and more. Split peas and lentils come like this too. In the 'Food Note' at the end of the chapter, I explain how I prepare dried beans and other pulses, and some ways I use them in recipes.

Vegetable versus animal proteins

Proteins are composed of amino acids, many of which are essential for body (and brain) health. Vegetable sources do not always contain all the necessary amino acids, although quinoa and buckwheat are among those that do. Animal sources of protein may bring the risk of higher cholesterol levels in certain circumstances. They are also connected to greater risks of developing some cancers. See the WCRF website for more information on the relationship between meat, fish and dairy consumption and certain cancer.

Industrialized meat production brings problems for animal welfare and affects the environment because it requires large volumes of water. It also results in the production of methane and causes pollution, as well as contributing to climate change. More information about these issues can be found at the Guardian's website, where you can find an article entitled 'The True Cost of Eating Meat'.

The current trend is to encourage less meat consumption because of these factors. A general comparison of different protein sources can be found on the *Medical News Today*'s website, where you can find an article entitled 'Which Is Better for Health'.

Carbohydrates

Rice and other grains, pasta, potatoes and breads seem to be the traditional providers of carbohydrate, although how they are processed and used depends on available resources, so geography and culture are significant. I remember working at a technology training centre for women years ago. The trainees came from a whole range of different backgrounds and so, of course, the children in the nursery reflected that diversity. One of the toys the children could play with was a plastic version of a basket of lots of differently shaped and coloured breads from many parts of the world. Sharing our different food cultures was one of the main ways (along with dancing) we would celebrate as a community.

Potatoes are probably one of my favourite foods and I serve them often, understanding that they are more nutritious if I leave the skins on, but not always doing that – traditional roast potatoes have to be peeled, to my way of thinking. . . . Eating pasta at home always reminds me of Italy, so, towards the end of the cooking time, I make a point of examining a piece of whatever type I have in the pan and checking its readiness very seriously, pulling at any long strands to judge the tension and maybe consulting others who will share it with me. When I was young, we only had rice pudding, which was a dessert. Nowadays, rice is a familiar savoury ingredient and many different types are easily available. People who are accustomed to cooking and eating rice seem to be able to keep the individual grains separate and glossy. My attempts often fall short of that but taste delicious nonetheless.

Carbs have a bit of a bad name at the moment, I think because of the sedentary lifestyle we have in the west. Nevertheless, they provide energy and are a necessary part of a healthy diet because they help create the right environment for the production of neurotransmitters in the brain (Geary, 2001). The healthiest way of eating carbs is to choose unrefined versions like brown rice and bread and pasta from wholemeal flours, and to eat the skin of the potatoes. I would also choose to use organically grown produce as much as possible, although the benefits of actually eating whole, fresh vegetables easily outweigh whether they are organic or not, if cost is an issue. More advice is available on the NHS' 'Live Well' website, where you can find more information on starchy foods and carbohydrates.

Fats

These are also separated into animal and vegetable versions. Some examples of animal fats are butter, ghee, lard, suet, cod liver oil and cheese. Vegetable fats include groundnut, olive and coconut oils. They are further categorized into saturated, poly-unsaturated and mono-unsaturated fats. Mostly, saturated fats are those that come from animals but, confusingly, there are many exceptions, for example, oily fish are unsaturated and coconut oil is saturated. Different types of nuts can have mainly poly-unsaturated or mono-unsaturated fats, which can add to the confusion.

The British Heart Foundation recommends choosing plant-based rather than animal-based sources of oil because of the effects saturated fats can have on blood circulation, which is an essential system supporting all the organs including (maybe especially) the brain. You can find more information on the British Heart Foundation's website, where you can find a section dedicated to sugar, salt and fat consumption.

In the past, fats have had a bad name in terms of nutrition because their calorific value is double that of proteins and carbohydrates. Nevertheless, they are important for a healthy diet because they provide essential fatty acids and support the absorption of some vitamins and minerals. They are particularly crucial for brain development in babies and children – breast milk is high in fat – and important for brain health throughout life.

> Fats matter a lot to emotional and mental health, with low levels in the diet being associated with symptoms that range from anxiety and depression to hyperactivity and schizophrenia.
>
> (Geary, 2001, p. 167)

Some areas for consideration are that palm oil, which is used widely in food production and packaging, has become controversial because its production contributes to deforestation, and therefore climate change, and the exploitation of workers. You can find more information on the WWF's website, where a resource is available called '8 things to know about palm oil'.

The type of spreads that are sold in plastic cartons need to be treated with caution because they are often highly processed and so less healthy than fats from more natural sources.

Dairy and eggs

I put these in a category by themselves because they are the products of animals, yet not animal flesh. Consequently, they are likely to be eaten by vegetarians, although definitely not by vegans. 'Dairy' includes milk, cream, cheese, butter, yoghurt, etc., and the various products in the category contain proteins, fats and other nutrients in differing proportions. For example, there is less fat in skimmed or semi-skimmed milk than there is in full fat, and more fat in cream and butter. Yoghurt comes in different versions, from full-fat to fat-free. At school I learned that cheese – which at that time was mainly cheddar – is one-third protein, one-third fat and one-third vitamins and minerals and water. Now that I have many more types of cheese freely available to me, the variation in the proportion of these nutrients becomes increasingly apparent. For instance, the higher fat content and intense flavour of stilton feels very different from a mouthful of fresh, light mozzarella. I can choose a variety that is appropriate for the season and appealing to my appetite. While artisanal cheese-making has become more common in recent years, so has the industrialization of milk production. The price the supermarkets will pay for milk has become so low that dairy farmers are forced into production methods that are sometimes controversial in order to remain in business. Please see the *Guardian*'s website to find an article entitled 'Dairy Scary: Public Farming'.

Eggs are a potentially healthy source of nutrients and can be a convenient and versatile choice of ingredient. I always choose the free-range organic option because I have the privilege of being able afford them and to have access to them, although even regular eggs are a good choice if resources are restricted. Omelettes are quick and easy suppers and hard-boiled eggs are brilliant for packed lunches because the shell provides ready-made packaging. For me, poached egg on toast or a soft-boiled egg with 'soldiers', which are made from a slice of buttered bread or toast cut into oblongs the right size to be dipped into the egg after cutting its top off, are some favourite 'comfort-foods'. More information about the issues involved in intensive egg production can be found on the CIWF's website.

Vitamins and minerals

The human body needs small amounts of a wide range of vitamins and minerals for proper functioning. Most of us would connect vitamin C with citrus fruits and maybe vitamin D with sunlight and currently the B vitamins, particularly B_6 and B_{12}, are being recognized as contributing to brain health because they are involved in the production of neurotransmitters (Geary, 2001). It is also generally known that calcium is connected with strong bones and teeth. Magnesium is perhaps less familiar, but it is important, being required for the production of essential fatty acids. Low levels of it are associated with anxiety, irritability and insomnia (Geary, 2001). It is found in leafy greens and nuts and I like to take hot baths with a cup of magnesium salts (also known as Epsom salts) thrown into the water and to absorb the benefits through my skin.

A list of all the vitamins and minerals needed for human health and wellbeing can be found on the NHS website.

The important thing about vitamins and minerals is that our bodies cannot produce them, so we have to consume them as a regular part of our diet. Oily fish, nuts, avocadoes, berries and broccoli are some of the foods that provide the nutrients we need. While many food supplements are available from specialist health shops and even supermarkets, probably the best way to ingest vitamins and minerals is from our food, and a balanced diet of all the food groups mentioned previously would provide a sufficient amount in the ordinary way.

Further information about important foods for brain (and general body) health can be found on *Medical News Today*'s website.

While writing this section, I was reminded about how important nuts are for nutrition – for example, walnuts are a rare non-animal provider of the omega-3 fatty acids that are essential for brain health (Geary, 2001). I try to follow a plant-based diet in the main, although I do eat fish and meat occasionally. Because of their high fat content, and therefore the calories they contain, I tended to avoid nuts. I am wary with avocado too, for a similar reason, but then sometimes I have a craving for it, and I can understand better now why that might be. Writing this section has made me change my food choices and as I pop a walnut half in my mouth, I can't help noticing how similar it looks to a brain, with its two hemispheres and winding structure.

Cuisines – communities and food

In the previous section, I separated food into different nutritional categories, but nobody actually eats that way. It is more usual, at least for me, to have a mix of foods on my plate at one time and to have different kinds of food at different times of day. For example, I might have porridge or eggs at breakfast, a salad with beans or egg or maybe a little cheese at lunchtime (except, of course, as I have already revealed, when I need the comfort of bread and butter). Supper would not be complete for me without potatoes, rice or pasta. Mostly, I would eat some concoction of vegetables, pulses, squashes or mushrooms that I discover as a recipe, or make up for myself depending on what's available in my kitchen, with my carbohydrate. Every few weeks I might have fish: hake or tuna or even, for a treat, traditional fried fish and chips from the local chip-shop. Sometimes I crave meat and then I salt and stretch a rib-eye steak – by this I mean that I bring the steak to room temperature, gently spread apart the meat with my hands and then season it with salt and pepper. Between touching the meat and reaching for the salt, I wash my hands really thoroughly. Then I wait for a while to let the salt soak in before cooking it quickly on a hot griddle, leaving it to settle for several minutes in a warm place after cooking, in order to let the juices run.

I rarely eat chicken but, as with other meat, I try and buy it from the person who produced it, mainly at farmers' markets. This is expensive, of course, but affordable as a rare indulgence. The seasonal veg and bags of beans and lentils I eat most of the time are relatively cheap. This diet has evolved over years and does involve time and forethought. In the past, I followed the tradition of 'meat and 2 veg' and, when I was working full-time with a young family, I would often buy convenience foods, so I understand the constraints of a busy life and pressures on time.

Although food from Europe and other parts of the world is freely available now, the traditional British diet is still deeply familiar to me. Living in Wales, I see sheep on the misty hillside, and cattle grazing on green fields, and bales of hay being driven around country lanes in late summer. It was a revelation to me to go to a sheep farm in Italy and notice the scrawnier, less woolly breeds that produce milk rather than meat and wool. Hard pecorino cheese and the creamy ricotta that is a by-product of the cheese-making process are eaten in that region, in contrast to the Sunday roast leg of lamb that is familiar to me.

The 'Mediterranean diet' is well recognized now as being one of the most healthy ways to eat. What is usually meant by this is lots of fruit vegetables and olive oil, some wine and little meat. Yet one of the things I notice about food in Italy (and I assume, in other countries around the Mediterranean) is how different much of what people eat is, depending on the type of agriculture the local land and climate can support and the different times of the year. In the middle of Sicily, in March, there were no tomatoes and no fish. But there were bitter greens, potatoes, chicken and the last of the citrus fruits in ornate, colourful bowls. It was only when I travelled to the coast that I could eat fish again, which I did with probably even greater relish for having missed it. So, the 'Mediterranean diet' covers a lot of possibilities!

As a result of my good fortune in being able to have had these kinds of experiences, I am a firm believer in eating what is local and seasonal, and wasting nothing (not always possible, unfortunately). Korn (2016, p. 4) also recommends that 'we should eat the types of food similar to the food our ancestors ate'. There are other healthy cuisines that have been recognized in the world, apart from the

Mediterranean diet, those in Japan and Norway, for example. Research findings from Professor Felice Jacka (2019, p. 39) have identified 'that people consuming diets traditional to their countries and cultures are less likely to have common mental disorders'. It seems that when people eat what is grown around them, they thrive (and so do the land and animals).

DNA and metabolism

Diet is personal, linked to the people and places that have produced us. A healthy balance of food choices for one person may not be suited to another. The genes we inherit are an important factor – our diets can be as unique as our DNA. The way our bodies process and assimilate the proteins, carbohydrates and fats in the food we eat influences our dietary choices. This is called metabolism or oxidization.

Leslie Korn (2016, p. 10) describes three nutritional types: the fast, slow or mixed oxidizer. She identifies the proportion of proteins, carbohydrates and fats that will suit bodies with each of the processing styles. I discovered I was a mixed oxidizer with my preference for a diet that comprises 30% protein, 40% carbohydrates and 30% fats. I find my senses draw me to this balance almost automatically: I can tell what I'm hungry for by the sensations in my eyes, mouth and stomach. More about body sensation, balance and regulation can be found in the next two chapters. More information about metabolism can be found on the NHS website's Live Well pages, under the tab 'metabolism and weight loss'.

The body reacts to lack of food by slowing down. In times of siege, crop failure and other periods of starvation, including deliberate under-eating, the body adapts by conserving energy. Available nutrients are directed away from the reproductive system, affecting the menstrual cycle, sexual drive and performance. Muscles are used as food; bones are depleted, vital organs shrink, and the heart and circulatory system becomes irregular, causing the sensation of being cold. The psychological effects accompanying these changes include depression, panic, obsessions, reduced thinking and decision-making capacity and disturbed sleep. Starving people may also have an experience of feeling fat (McKenna, 2020). Disordered eating is discussed more fully in the next chapter. More information may be found on the Sedig's website, under 'physical and psychological effects of the starvation syndrome'.

Chapter summary

We obtain the nourishment that we need in order to live a healthy life (or any kind of life at all) from food. Our diets and lives are also interdependent with the food environment in which we are embedded. This is both historical (our families) and geographical (where we came from). How and where our food is grown, and how much awareness we have of it in our daily lives, is so intrinsic we may have to bring it purposely into awareness to understand its impact. Where and how we obtain our food can either contribute to or detract from general wellbeing and enjoying a truly satisfying life.

Activities

Please consider the following questions. This may involve thinking about them, meditating on them or making a piece of free-flowing, uncensored writing, similar to those in a personal journal.

2.1 How would you describe your own food culture?
2.2 Thinking of a client, would you share a food culture, or would your experiences be very different?
2.3 Is your own food culture the same as that of the society in which you live, or different?

Personal reflection

Written by Kevin Williamson RNutr (Public Health), a Consultant Nutritionist supporting the nutritional needs of those with mental health issues, and Head of Service for an NHS Trust research team in the North of England. He is studying for a PhD in how nutrition supports psychosis symptom management.

As a student nutritionist I was always interested in mental health. Before studying nutrition I had worked on some local authority policies to support mental health at the workplace. I was delighted when, after graduating, I successfully secured a new post to develop a nutritional care service for people experiencing psychosis.

For me, nutrition is so basal, it infiltrates everything. It may sound trite to use the old adage 'we are what we eat', but physiologically speaking it's true. Every cellular reaction that has taken place, is taking place or will ever take place involves a huge array of different nutritional compounds. These of course come from what we eat and drink. Food though is so much more and in terms of our wellbeing, food has a social and cultural connection to us; food is related to traditions and memories and food is something we need to have a healthy relationship with. If we have an unhealthy relationship with food, we can't treat it like drugs or alcohol and just avoid it. Fundamentally, food should bring us joy and pleasure.

It's clear to me though that everyone, or almost everyone, struggles to have a healthy relationship with food at some point or another in their lives. For some, the struggle remains a continuous one that affects them throughout life. I think though that this struggle is made so much greater for those experiencing mental health difficulties, partly due perhaps to the physiological or biochemical processes related to the issues, or maybe due to the change in lifestyle that can accompany mental health struggles.

In my years working in mental health services I saw many people who were really interested and engaged in the concept of nutrition as part of mental healthcare. There were some who included nutrition and diet as part of their recovery, and also as part of their recovery plan. There were several examples of individuals who increased their dietary knowledge and improved their dietary habits through increasing consumption of whole foods, fruit, vegetables and oily fish and drastically reduced their consumption of processed foods. In addition to this though,

*I saw some individuals who used diet and nutrition to change their social cir-
cumstance, with one individual who had previously struggled to leave the house,
hosting cooking classes for the local community. There were also others who used
newly acquired cooking skills to 'have friends round for food'. This social aspect
of food feels like an important part of mental wellbeing.*

*Whilst there is a firm evidence base for the physiological importance of nutri-
tion and a lot of anecdotal knowledge within mental health services of the importance of food, diet and nutrition aren't at the top of the research or care agenda.
I feel strongly that there needs to be a greater emphasis on the connection between
food, health and wellbeing among health professionals.*

Food note

'This week's beans'

I usually soak and cook a pan of beans every week, to accompany the contents of
my veg box. I choose the different varieties in turn: chickpeas, red kidneys, borlotti or butter beans, and others if I find a recipe I want to try. I pour the amount
I think I need into a big metal bowl and cover well with cold water. For me, 250
grammes is about the right amount but I don't measure particularly accurately,
I just tip the chosen beans into my familiar vessel. The amount you need is likely
to be different, so some experimenting may be needed. After about 24 hours,
I drain and rinse the beans, noticing how much they have swollen, and put them
in a big saucepan, covering them well with cold water (no salt) and bringing to
the boil. Keep watching as the pan heats. The beans need to stay at boiling point
long enough to destroy any unhelpful chemicals, including those that cause wind
in the body (about 40 minutes). Conversely, they need to boil in a tranquil enough
way so that the little individuals remain whole, and firm enough to use in recipes.
Observation and practice are the best guides, as with many things. As they boil,
some scum might appear on the surface of the water. Skim this off with a table-
spoon and discard it. When you think they are nearly done, scoop one out and try
it. If it is soft, but still has firmness and integrity, they are ready, so turn off the
heat. When the pan has cooled, I transfer the beans **and the cooking liquid** into
a large plastic storage box and keep it in the fridge for the week, scooping out the
amount I need with a big, holey spoon as I go along.

References

Geary, A. (2001) *The food and mood handbook.* London: Thorsons.
Jacka, F. (2019) *Brainchanger.* Great Britain: Yellow Kite.
Korn, L. (2016) *Nutrition essentials for mental health.* New York: Norton.
Leyse-Wallace, R. (2008) *Linking nutrition to mental health.* Lincoln, NE: iUniverse.
McKenna, B. (2020) *Food and mood: A guide to mental health.* Belfast: Course Handout.

3 Roots

Factors underlying relationships with food

Introduction

Each of us has our own particular relationship with food, and the families and society in which we live have theirs too. When relationships with food, either individual or societal, tip too much out of balance, it can result in what is recognized as disordered eating. This affects general health and wellbeing and also has an impact on the services that are provided to address the associated challenges.

For individuals, a disordered relationship with food can be a threat to life and is always a threat to contentment and wellbeing. Over time, unhealthy food choices can have physical, mental and emotional consequences, maybe even spiritual ones for some people. Human beings are complex organisms, and while our distress may become apparent in our bodies, it affects our minds and emotions too. Psychological and emotional distress can also become physical distress, leading to conditions like chronic fatigue and pain that seems to have no apparent physical cause (Panksepp and Biven, 2012).

While mood and emotional state may not be directly related with food, they are likely to affect appetite and food choices. We are also increasing our understanding of the direct relationship between what we eat and how we feel (Jacka, 2019).

The experiences we have in our families of origin are the foundation for the sense of wellbeing or unease with which we approach our lives, including our relationships with food, and influence how much resilience we have for dealing with the inevitable challenges we meet. In our families, we learn about relationships with other people and with the variety of other resources we need to keep us alive.

Our bodies, instincts and intuitions, emotions and thoughts are all involved in maintaining mental health. We need to explore all these aspects in order to form a picture of what mental health means for us. Each of us is a unique individual, so how we experience mental health is particular to ourselves. Naturally, it is likely we will notice similarities with other family members, and with other humans in general, because of the experiences we have in common.

While this book is meant as a guide for people who facilitate others around health issues, it is also an invitation for all of us to be our own 'health professional'. By doing so, we can feel some agency around achieving or maintaining what we experience as mental health and wellbeing.

DOI: 10.4324/9781003172161-4

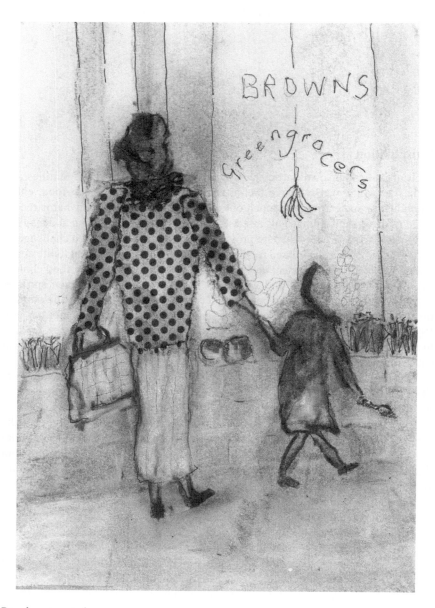

Deeply connected

Chapter structure

The issues being discussed in this chapter may be difficult and painful for some readers. In order to make the material easier to digest, I am dividing it into three parts.

Part One begins with an exploration of some of the kinds of relationships with food that human beings experience, including those categorized as eating disorders. Some of the consequences of disordered eating patterns for individuals and the wider society are described here, and a 'Personal Reflection' offers further insight around the subjective experience of difficult relationships with food. Then there will be a pause and a chance to draw breath and reflect.

In **Part Two**, we begin to understand the deep connections between attitudes to food and attitudes to life in general. When we explore how we regulate our food intake we are at the same time exploring how we relate generally – with other people and with the world around us. In order to begin to address some of the issues underlying challenging relationships with food, it becomes necessary to understand what it means to be human and to be living in the world. This is important because it is the basis for mental health. Being human is multi-faceted and involves our bodies, emotions and thoughts, and also the effect of our upbringing, culture and way of life.

The faculties we have to signal our needs around food are appetite, hunger, satisfaction, pleasure, discomfort, disgust and others. These are words that relate to sensations we experience in our bodies. Actual body experience takes place in the world, where there is gravity, air, nature and other living beings, particularly other humans. Most of what we call our experience is interaction with the world in which we participate – a constant negotiation between what we recognize as 'me' and what we perceive as 'other'. Breathing is the most obvious and enduring manifestation of this interconnectedness, and food is another.

Part Three offers a glimpse into the therapy room by means of case studies that reveal how some people resolve the issues that may be troubling them. If you have taken in enough previously in the chapter, then this section can be skipped.

Part one – relationships with food

It is necessary to eat to stay alive but, for each of us, our relationship with eating often turns out to be a negotiation. We experience the beginning of the development of that relationship very early on in life, shaped by our parents or carers. People come from different backgrounds and have a whole range of early life experiences. Maybe this is a reflection of my own experience, but I believe that, to all intents and purposes, we receive food and care as the same thing. Not all mothers and babies know the rapture of successful breast feeding. Feeds, and later meals, can have a mixed emotional and nutritional atmosphere. Relationships with food can be fraught and, as we grow up, we are exposed to increasing expectations about what we achieve, how we act and how we look, so it is little wonder that eating can be problematical.

Some of us may negotiate food intake in a way that seems comfortable enough, others may look like they are managing reasonably well but pay a price for their slim figures. Still others might fail to manage the negotiation effectively at all and then cannot hide the effects of that. I was a fat child when most other people were thin, so my size was what people saw and therefore it defined me, and I hated that. Extreme thinness often reveals the existence of an anorexic or bulimic relationship but, then again, not always. It is possible to be very thin and not have a disordered relationship with food. Each of us somehow decides for ourselves whether our diet and body weight are comfortable or problematic for us, although we can be affected by the expectations and judgements of others, and the cultures within which we live.

Eating patterns connected with extremes of over- or underweight, combined with associated emotional or psychological responses, are what society calls 'eating disorders'. When I was training, I was required to do placements at some NHS establishments where mental health problems were treated. I had the opportunity then to speak to one of the leading experts on eating disorders at that time. I was overweight myself, and conscious of it, although neither of us mentioned the fact. She began our discussion by telling me that the main eating disorders were classified as anorexia, bulimia and overeating, but that they were concerned with treating only anorexia and bulimia. I asked her why and, after a moment's thought she replied that it was because anorexia and bulimia were life-threatening.

These days, the threat to life posed by overeating is much better recognized but, back then, I only sat, silent and uncomfortable, with the knowing that the consequences of overeating felt to me like they were indeed life-threatening. I had a very dear friend who died a few years ago from cancer. She was also a therapist and one of her special interests was how people experience shame. I think I was a bit blasé back then because I responded quite casually to something she said with 'People don't die of shame though, do they'.

'Yes, they do'. She responded immediately and vehemently, and I believed her. Many years later, I was talking to someone else, I think it was at a Weight Watchers meeting, about dieting. She said to me, 'People don't die of hunger though, do they'. My immediate response was 'Yes, they do'. This echo of the previous conversation really taught me something about how hunger, shame and other sensations and emotions can feel connected and similarly life-threatening to humans. This may be because of our absolute dependence on our carers as babies when any withdrawal of love (or food) is soon lethal at that stage.

It is very possible, of course, to die of hunger. People do it every day. I know from my own experience that it is also possible to feel hunger and to feel like you might die from it, even when the next meal is not so very far away. I also know from speaking to others that it is possible to feel like there is a threat to life from having to eat. I have seen people look very frightened by a plate of pastries being brought in with the coffee at a meeting or an invitation to go to lunch with a group of relative strangers.

I have felt sometimes that I needed to conceal my relish for food, but there were situations when I felt comfortable enough not to have to do it. I remember standing in the queue for a lunch buffet at a holistic centre where I was taking a course and saying to the person next to me, whom I knew quite well, how good the food looked. She was an attractive, svelte woman and she told me how much she envied my ability to relish the food and that it was something denied to her.

Eating disorders

Most of us will be familiar with these conditions and probably know people who have been affected by them or else have experienced them ourselves. They are defined separately because they categorize two distinct types of relationship with eating, although it seems to me each person has their own particular, individual experience. I describe my understanding of both of them in the following. The NHS website has more information and advice (www.nhs.uk/conditions/anorexia/symptoms/)

I know there are other eating disorders besides these two. Specialist sources of information and advice may be accessed here: https://eating-disorders.org.uk.

If you are concerned about yourself or a family member, then the best port of call is your own general practitioner (GP).

Anorexia

People I have worked with may say something like, 'I wasn't in control of much, but I could be in control of that', or else they might be striving for 'perfection' because they are involved in sport, or dance, or they may not even know why losing weight became so essential at a particular time of their lives, sometimes discovering the reason for it in our work together. The kind of relationship with food that is associated with anorexia is that of eating as little as possible, often choosing low calorie food (or food that somehow feels 'safe'), aiming to lose weight and achieve some kind of ideal size. Unfortunately, part of what may happen is that people's perception of an ideal size becomes distorted, which is how someone who is very thin may say 'I look fat'. When I work with people who have this kind of process, I anticipate that it may be very difficult for them to accept emotional and psychological nourishment too, and we may explore this together. I also become acutely aware of my own body size and how I might be perceived. I remember years ago, before I lost weight, working with the mother of a young woman who had been diagnosed with anorexia, and noticing her extreme discomfort at talking about these things with me. I believed I felt comfortable to explore them with her (having worked on the issues in my own therapy) and tried to convey it both directly and indirectly. Nevertheless, she ended sessions relatively quickly and I was left to reflect in supervision on what might have been out-of-awareness for me with that client at the time.

Bulimia

The words that are generally used about a bulimic process are 'binge and purge'. These little verbs seem to convey the extremities of people's experience very well. A number of times, people asking to work with me have told me they 'are bulimic' (their choice of words) but it may be a very long time before they are able to disclose to me exactly how they regulate their hunger and food intake, and I accept this as the dynamic of their relationship with food being reflected in their current style of interaction with me. People with this issue may seem attractive and successful, but I have heard about vomit being hidden in biscuit tins under the bed. And I have actually heard a well-dressed woman in her thirties being sick in the toilet cubicle next to mine in a hotel after a wedding breakfast at which we were both guests.

Overeating

I believe that, in the UK today, it is very easy to overeat. By this, I mean to eat more calories than our bodies need to fuel the activities we undertake. It is probably less easy to eat a diet that provides the nutrients we need to live a satisfying life and keep our bodies at a weight that is healthy for us. As briefly discussed in Chapter 1, part of the reason for this is that emphasis is placed on offering food for sale as cheaply as possible. When processed food is cheaper than buying fresh vegetables, it is tempting to take what feels like an easy way out. For families experiencing poverty, it is almost impossible to exercise any choice other than to buy what is cheap and available. In general, even when there are children, it is more common for both partners to go out to work now, outsourcing cooking by choosing ready meals and takeaways, rather than dividing the roles of income generation and household upkeep. I discuss food policy more fully in Chapter 5 and the impact of gender, race and class in Chapter 6.

It is more common than it was for people to be overweight, so maybe less stigma is involved. Although maybe not, because of fashion industry, media and social media representations that so often portray extreme thinness as being desirable. In these circumstances, attitudes and feelings are likely to be fluid, conflicted and even more complex than previously, potentially creating more stress for the individual.

I have noticed that overweight often runs in families, it certainly did in mine. I was encouraged to eat as much as possible. Whether this is because my mother remembered rationing from the war, or because she had experienced stillbirth with a previous child and wanted to do everything she possibly could to keep me alive, or that she confused food with love, or that she didn't know what else to do with a screaming child. . . . As I grew up, I would count how many roast potatoes she had piled on to my father's plate at Sunday dinner, and used to want the same amount. I wanted as much as he had, but I never got it. Somehow, the right to food seemed an important entitlement. I don't think either parent liked to see me fat even though, all the while, they pressed food upon me. It seems significant to me that I was only able to lose weight after both my parents had died. I have heard other people talk about a hunger that could not be satisfied (see the Personal Reflection at the end of the chapter for a description of this kind of process). I don't think my experience is like that, although if I were to be offered a superpower, I would choose to be able to eat and drink as much as I like and not put on weight.

Other impacts of an uneasy relationship with food

Physical impact

As discussed earlier, death is the most extreme physical outcome of an uneasy relationship with food. This could involve someone literally starving themselves to death. It could also be an outcome of years of bad food choices, beginning in childhood, or the impact of carrying extremely excessive weight on the organs of the body.

Some common diseases currently connected with diet are type 2 diabetes, cancer and heart attack and stroke. Type 2 diabetes, a condition where sugar levels in the body can no longer be regulated effectively, is on the increase in the UK and is understood as being connected with an unhealthy diet. See www.diabetes.org.uk/professionals/position-statements-reports/statistics.

Cancer is connected with unhealthy diets and particularly with ultra-processed foods: more information is available on the NHS website by following links to ultra-processed food and cancer.

Heart attacks and strokes are associated with too much saturated fat: www.bhf.org.uk/informationsupport/heart-matters-magazine/nutrition/sugar-salt-and-fat/saturated-fat-animation.

There can be more subtle consequences of a difficult relationship with food, for example, the vomiting associated with bulimia can negatively affect the balance of alkalinity in the body and so cause harm over time (Geary, 2001, p. 26). I think it is likely that I will eventually die from my lifelong food choices. Maybe in Western society, many of us will, and perhaps that feels more 'civilized' than succumbing to disease, being broken by harsh physical work as my grandparents were or attacked by a wild animal.

Early warning

Being overweight for much of my life has put pressure on my joints, the consequence of which is becoming more apparent as I grow older. Other people have to take medication for cholesterol or high blood pressure. These are some of the not (yet) as serious physical outcomes of bad food choices.

Nutrition and mental health expert Leslie Korn identifies inflammation of the body and brain as an early warning sign of potential future issues. Inflammation is a natural response to ingesting anything that is toxic for the body (including environmental pollution) and also to physical or emotional injury. Swelling of the joints and reddening of the skin are some visible signs. It is meant to occur when needed, resolve the problem and then subside. If the stressors continue to be experienced consistently, then inflammation can become chronic, which means the reaction of the body's immune system never fully switches off. Along with the physical consequences, like pain and the possibility of developing more serious conditions, the substances secreted by the body in response to inflammation-related stressors can harm nerve cells and cause feelings of depression (Korn, 2016, p. 3).

Naturopathic physician Anne Procyk (2018) recognizes that chronic inflammation can affect the autoimmune system and slow down the healing process. Any injuries that seem to be taking an inappropriately long time to heal may indicate the presence of inflammation. Overwhelming physical or emotional trauma may be a trigger for inflammation. Certain food groups, wheat dairy and the 'night-shade' family (aubergines, tomatoes, peppers and potatoes), may also be contributing factors. Other aspects connected with inflammation include stress, poor diet, lack of exercise and sleep, smoking and toxic substances (Korn, 2016, p. 3). All these are very familiar aspects of our current lifestyles.

Eating a diet rich in green vegetables helps against inflammation as do the spices turmeric, ginger and saffron.

More information is available at: www.medicalnewstoday.com/articles/248423# chronic-or-acute.

Mental and emotional impact

Whatever our current physical challenges may be, we are exposed to mental and emotional consequences that are equally distressing. We are whole beings and we experience our existence holistically, although the mental or physical symptoms may each be highlighted at particular times and at different stages of life.

Clear links have been identified between diet and depression, Alzheimer's, schizophrenia, post-traumatic stress disorder and autism (Korn, 2016). These conditions have specific names that distinguish them from other experiences because a commonality has been found with how sufferers experience them. Yet subjective, direct experience of distress is actually what happens when any of us succumbs to these or other less specific ailments.

Health, society and lifestyle impact

I was born a few years after the NHS was founded. Children with leg braces or strange deformities were a common sight. Everybody had bad teeth. An older client of mine described her experience of being a child patient on the actual day the NHS began. She had previously been receiving treatment for appendicitis, which her family was having to pay for. From that day on, it was free. Even 50 years later, she looked at me with wonder as she described that moment. More than 70 years of medical care that is free at the point of access, along with growing affluence, means that people have become physically healthier.

Even after the 2020 pandemic, in the west, the physical risks we have to negotiate to stay alive have been declining, and treatments are available for many of our ailments, including the effects of those brought on by our lifestyle choices about food, smoking and exercise. Nevertheless, there is no treatment for consistently unhealthy food choices and public awareness of the impact of the way our food system works in the UK has been growing. I return to this in Chapter 5.

Summary

Our relationships with food begin to be formed early on. When they are problematic, they affect every aspect of our lives. Beginning to address the issues connected with them involves giving attention to all the facets of our being. Environmental factors, like the kind of food that is available, are also relevant.

Personal reflection – food and I

Written by Mary Hughes. Artist and Coaching Supervisor. Wales.

"Suda makhan?" (Have you eaten?) is what every Malaysian will ask having greeted you with their heart open and called down blessings for your health and prosperity. Food is that important as a cultural element, an expression of inclusive generosity, a holy thing presented as a beautiful gift. I grew up with balanced flavours, the poetic language of sour, salt, sweet, umami, fat and heat composed to perfection, however humbly, and always full of integrity for the spirit of place.

For a little girl in the mid-twentieth century just arrived from an entire life lived in what is now Malaysia, it was bewildering. Mum did her best, but I gagged on porridge and wept over pies as she (a natural saint) endured the adjustments from South East Asia to North West Europe. The greatest of all of these for me being about my palate, my digestive system and familiar tastes; the savour of flavour.

"Oi, Blackie, where d'you think you're going?" The prefect shouted. "It's dinner time, now!". An hour later I was shaking with fear before a plate of mince and mash with a bowl of pink custard on one side and a sharp-tongued teacher on the other. My first day in a British school and a lifelong aftertaste. . . . That evening I was in detention accompanied by the same plate of cold, congealed food. In Malaysia, to be punished for a food-related reason would have been shocking, especially if meted out to a child. There's always a flavour to tempt, a texture to revel in and a sensation to invoke, so why beat a single drum when you could use other instruments? I was dark haired and the remnants of 10 years under the tropical sun staining my skin meant I was known as, "Blackie". This didn't affect me, in fact I felt better because it might mean I was somehow not quite as blotchy, red-nosed or catarrhal as my new classmates. I shivered in itchy jumpers throughout the entire summer and the in-doors, dusty way of life was suffocating and smelly, I accepted it because my parents seemed so happy to be back. But the food! The soft, greasy, milky, over-salty tasteless mush of it!

I know now how much school dinners meant to some of the kids and their families, but they were utterly uncompromising when it came to a process of cultural adjustment. It felt like a one-size-fits-all approach boiled up in the war years, unseasoned ever since and not a thought about perfume, taste or how it made you feel. Looking back, it seemed (as, to be fair, it may have needed to be) an economically determined attempt to keep us alive and warm with a very minimal choice of ingredients and generalised assumptions about what the average child would eat on a strict budget. Food, in short, was culturally a very, very different place from the hot, humid, flavoursome land I had known. The biggest evil was waste which was quite simply, a crime deserving of direct, corporal punishment. And, at school, my body was pun-ished and with it my mind and my heart. I never had detention for bad school-work or bad behaviour, just for not eating school food.

In Malaysia food was all about celebrating and a joy, never a duty or a solely commercial concern. Food was never difficult; carefully made and fin-ished, it might be complex but always a matter of revered skill and attention. There was an accompanying orchestra of fruits, nuts and vegetables playing symphonies in my mouth. The recipe for British culture was served up on the plate of duty and came back again and again until you ingested it; or learned how to appear to do so. Cultural value was (may still be) judged primarily on surface behaviour, so I learned how to present my surface. This meant swallowing chunks without tasting, shovelling the drier bits into something that could be thrown away and spitting out the chewy stuff down the toilet. To rid myself of the weight of noncompliance and inevitable comeuppance, I lied and cheated. Food avoidance taught me that a sure way to survive without having to explain all the time why I should be entitled to do so, meant to live a falsehood. To pretend to be eating the same things at the same table with everyone else became a philosophy applied beyond eating. I developed coping mechanisms to manage the stress induced. I went through phases of anorexia, bulimia, low self-esteem, insomnia and the sort of anxiety that turned blood to bile triggered by any accusation of not belonging. But I also learned with huge expertise to keep it all hidden, always hidden even, eventually, from that supposed place of safety, my family. Falsehood buried deep under falsehood. She's 'naturally thin', 'allergic to dairy' and 'a worrier'; the 'What-She-Is-Like' narrative I spun to spare others the job of looking any harder (and in case of what they might find). The table-top of my life was laid out neatly and could belong, but the kitchen of my life wouldn't have passed any hygiene test.

I can't remember when I actually managed to adjust, but I do remember it had much to do with reorganising my own metaphorical kitchen, realising I had a palate of my own with character. Moreover, some shared it. Like the French friend who gave me gloriously ripe, runny Camembert, the Italian mother of a boyfriend who made delicious, simple pasta with flavoursome olive oil and fresh garlic and the Jamaican cafe with gorgeous spicy bean stews. Then the joy of my first Indian restaurant where I ate with relish what the cool kids gagged on. I suppose I found others from that great, big place beyond called, 'Abroad' and through their food found some form of belong-ing. OK, 'Blackie' had now faded into 'Whitey' but my soul never bleached! I don't think my tastes changed, I just had to find ways of integrating them because until I did, no-one else made the effort to integrate me. What I notice now, however, is how that became easier when the insistence that I conform was slackened off and conformity itself became somewhat passé. As British culture changed in the later twentieth century, much of it thanks to a diversity of peoples bringing their food as well as their philosophies with them, so orthodoxies were challenged. The only eternity I know is change and human change is a rich recipe, spiced with culture, new flavours added all the time.

Pause

Take a moment here to connect with your body and notice what is happening.

Notice without judgement and with compassion if necessary.

Become conscious of your breath.

Food and sense of self are so connected, our emotional responses to exploring these things can be powerful.

It is possible to heal from disordered eating and even from actual eating disorders. The next section begins an exploration of that, which continues in the next chapter.

Check if you have had enough for now and need to take a rest and come back later when your appetite is stimulated again. Otherwise, here is the next part of the journey.

Part two – beginning to address difficult relationships with food and the challenge of being human

An unhealthy relationship with food, whether experienced as mainly connected with the body or with the mind, may lead to despair, fear, anger, guilt, shame, blaming and remorse and perhaps a vicious cycle of harmful behaviours. Self-esteem can be so seriously challenged that self-harming behaviour is the only possible response in the circumstances. Hitting, biting, cutting and burning are extreme physical manifestations, but there are many more subtle, hidden ones. Being involved in extreme or dangerous sports can be an outcome of self-loathing. Promiscuous, unsafe sexual behaviour can indicate low self-worth. Ignoring body sensations like thirst or the need to visit the bathroom may indicate an out-of-awareness desire to deny or punish the body. Self-isolation and restricting engagement with life is another possible outcome. Many clients bring these issues to therapy. Caught up in overwhelming life situations, it is difficult (and probably unnecessary) to distinguish between thoughts, emotions and body sensations – every bit of us just feels awful. While they dynamically interact with each other all the time, it can be helpful to consider the role of thoughts and emotions, and something about relational styles separately as a way increasing awareness and becoming more effective in our work with clients.

Thoughts

In Western society, we tend to prioritize our thinking, intellect and decision-making capacity over the sensations in our bodies. Perhaps Descartes can be attributed with separating mind and body in this way. 'Our world is a giant mechanism not unlike a clock. . . . [I]t runs on the principles of mechanics, and our science is mechanistic in principle' is how philosopher Norman Melchert sums up Descartes' view (2014, p. 352). In the twenty-first century, this dualism – the splitting of mind and body, seeing the body as a type of machine governed by the all-important brain – is being challenged. Philosopher Daniel Dennett has coined the term 'cartesian theatre' almost as a parody of the kind of thinking that leads us to imagine a control centre in the brain where all our sensory processes are analysed and a plan of action is formed in response (see https://en.wikipedia.org/wiki/Cartesian_theater). There are many clips on YouTube in which Dennett affirms that a cartesian theatre view of being is flawed, that the reality is less centralized and more organic than Descartes imagined.

In Chapter 1 of his book 'The Mind-Gut Connection' (2016), American physician Emeran Mayer examines this mechanistic world view and how it has influenced approaches to healing in the west. He offers pointers for compelling alternative possibilities, involving more holistic approaches, that may contribute to resolving the crises in healthcare he identifies.

Our large brains provide us with imagination and allow us to run what-if scenarios in our heads. Left unchecked, our minds can expose us to all sorts of possibilities, and sometimes that means we can cause ourselves great suffering. When I watch my daughter's springer spaniel curled up in her basket, I see from her reposeful state that she is not thinking about whether she caught the ball well enough in the park earlier, that she isn't wondering whether she has enough dry biscuits for supper or worrying that her arthritis might get worse. She is just there, lying with her throat resting comfortably on her front paws. When her breathing changes, and I notice that she has fallen asleep, her slight twitches and whimpers tell me that she is dreaming, but that is a different thing.

The success of humans as a species comes from our ability to theorize, extrapolate and plan, to discuss our ideas with one another, and consult historical learning in books and, increasingly now, the internet. We are able to use our minds to think about/imagine experiences that our bodies have not enacted, although as we do think about them our bodies are likely to respond as if they are actually taking place. But the downside of this crucial attribute is that our thoughts can run away with themselves without our noticing. To describe it that way sounds like separating the self, our whole being, into parts that squabble and interact, a bit like characters in the cartesian theatre might. Subjectively, I believe, we do experience it that way. Certainly, my subjective experience is like that. We use terms like the Buddhist expression 'monkey mind' (https://en.wikipedia.org/wiki/Monkey_mind) to capture the nature of it. The ancients understood the dynamic well. This beautiful prayer comes from the yoga tradition:

> May students come to me from far and near,
> Like a river flowing all the year.
> May I be enabled to guide them all
> To train their senses and still their minds.
> May this be my wealth, may this be my fame.
>   (Taittiriya Upanishad. V. 2–3)

Although I have practised yoga for many years, I don't consider myself an expert. Yet I find myself often exploring how to train our senses and still our minds with the people with whom I work. It seems like an essential life skill to me. You can find the whole text this piece was taken from here:

https://holybooks.com/the-taittiriya-upanishad-the-complete-pdf/.

Still in the Hindu tradition, the great elephant-headed god Ganesh is always depicted with a mouse. Some images show the mouse pulling the chariot in which the god rides. The absurdity of a great elephant-headed god being pulled around by a tiny rodent is thought by some to mirror the way that humans can allow themselves to be driven by their thoughts, to their detriment. We forget that we are much more than just our thoughts (www.biodiversityofindia.org/index. php?title=Why_Lord_Ganesha_has_a_mouse_as_his_vehicle).

Naturally, our thinking capacity and the knowledge we possess are an important resource and do help us to make good choices. Much of Chapter 2 is information, meant to increase knowledge and extend and maybe reorientate ways of thinking about specific topics and to hone decision making in situations where they are relevant, particularly with clients. But to really know how to regulate food choices, and life choices in general, we need to rely on signals from our bodies, emotions and even our spiritual natures too. I will suggest possible ways of approaching this integration in the next chapter.

Internalizing the relational environment

The Transactional Analysis approach to psychotherapy, whose founder was Eric Berne, suggests that our internal processes can be organized into three 'ego states', which are called parent, adult and child. Berne defines ego states as: 'coherent systems of thought and feeling manifested by corresponding patterns of behaviour' (Berne, 1988, p. 11). They evolve over time. The relational process we experience as children with our carers results in the creation of a notional internal parent in our minds. By the time we physically become adults, this internalized parent performs a similar kind of role to that of our actual parents or carers, either nurturing or punishing. To complement this, we also create a notional internal child that can be either spontaneous and lovable, or suppressed into compliance with parental expectations. A notional adult ego state develops that can (hopefully) mediate choicefully in the internal parent-child dynamic and generally encounter the world capably and with confidence. The kind of activity that operates in the mind can often parallel actual early experience. If that was good enough, then the ecology is relatively tranquil, and if not, then the voice of a cruel, highly critical or dismissive parent can often be reproduced in the constant activity of the human mind.

This theory also works at an interpersonal level. We may communicate with others from one or other of the ego states, maybe preferring one in particular most of the time, or perhaps changing, depending on circumstances. We also respond to the quality of the ego state from which another person is communicating. Does your internal parent respond to the internal child of the other person? Or vice versa? Are your interactions mainly adult to adult? Of course, there is no particular right or wrong way of using this. Having flexibility and finding what works best in the current circumstances is what can help us towards the outcomes we want to achieve, particularly with clients.

Creating catastrophe

Many of my clients describe how they lie in bed at night, sleepless for hours, going over potential possibilities in their minds. Heart-pounding and vigilant, they suffer failure, loss and destitution. This is another example of the ability our minds have to imagine situations that have not actually occurred. Having begun to think about something, our emotional responses become engaged, and then our bodies begin to release adrenalin and sleep becomes impossible. This happens in the daytime too. How many of us experience the lurch of panic 'I've lost my car keys!' only to find them in the other pocket . . . Portuguese neurologist Antonio Damasio observes:

> Emotions occur in one of two types of circumstances. The first type of cir-
> cumstance takes place when the organism processes certain objects or situ-
> ations with one of its sensory devices. . . . The second type of circumstance
> occurs when the mind of an organism conjures up from memory certain
> objects and situations.
>
> (Damasio, 2000, p. 56)

Emotional and body reactions can follow thought, but this is not always the best way. Different approaches have grown up over time to help us to manage our thought processes. I have already mentioned Buddhism and yoga, but there is also meditation and the practice of mindfulness, which can help disentangle us from constant thinking and support increased emotional awareness. See https:// en.wikipedia.org/wiki/Mindfulness for more information.

When my clients start mentioning that they are experiencing unruly thought processes that keep them awake at night, I share my own strategies for dealing with this when it happens to me. Which, being a natural human process, of course, it does. I like to begin by focusing on my breathing. This immediately distracts me from whatever scenarios I am constructing in my mind and brings me back to my body in the present moment. I notice that I am safe, warm and comfortable, and reassure myself that the things I'm imagining haven't actually happened and probably won't. Even if they do, I would probably be able to deal with it. I call this internal dialogue self-talk, and some kind of reassuring verbal message, even though it comes from myself (or maybe from a symbolic internalized 'other' like a parent, teacher, therapist or friend), seems to help. I notice how the mattress is supporting my body and allow myself to broaden and relax. I like to keep my focus on my body and breath to stop myself re-entering the maelstrom and soon I fall asleep. The traditional way is to count sheep and I suppose that might do just as well.

Emotions

Fear, anger, sadness, love, awe, despair, frustration, compassion, loss, loneliness, shame, guilt, delight, etc., all these are what we recognize as emotional experiences. Mostly, I become aware that I am experiencing an emotion because I notice distinctive, familiar sensations in my body that feel essential to my sense of being alive in the world. The heat of anger, the damp weight of sadness, the adrenalin rush of fear, all these and more I recognize. I know that others are familiar with them too and that each of us understands intuitively when another person is experiencing them (Carter, 2019). They occur in relation to 'other', mostly other people.

A rich emotional range helps us feel truly alive, but that is not always available to everyone. In our families of origin, some emotions are more acceptable than others. Our individual access to emotion may be dependent on our gender or place in the family. For example (and it may seem like a cliché), boys used to be discouraged from crying and girls from being angry. It will be interesting to see how less fixed gender expectations affect the next generation. More nuanced dynamics that I have seen very commonly are when it is a child's role to keep the peace in the family or to care for mother. We learn to suppress unwelcome emotions, holding them unexpressed in our bodies for years, maybe a whole lifetime.

Emotions and the mind

To help practitioners become more skilful in understanding and working with our own and our clients' emotional expression, it may be helpful to know more about how emotions have evolved. In 'The Archaeology of Mind: Neuroevolutionary Origins of Human Emotions', Panksepp and Biven (2012) offer an interesting, new understanding. They differentiate between emotions that are connected with more primitive (earlier) subcortical (secondary level) brain development and those that are connected with later (tertiary level) frontal cortex development. They define the earlier emotions as: Seeking; Rage; Fear; Lust; Care; Grief and Play. I am using capital letters because I am following the conventions of the book, which attempts to differentiate them slightly from the way we might define them ordinarily. While the range they have identified fits with my subjective experience, I was surprised by the inclusion of Seeking. Briefly, the authors describe a state of going out into the world to find what we need. To understand this characteristic as connected with emotion rather than cognition is comforting to me somehow.

One important aspect of this work is that the brains of other mammals have developed in the identical way. This means that the squirrel hunting for acorns in my garden has the same connection to the activity emotionally as I do to my experience of seeking work, or interesting new ideas, or something delicious for my own supper. I observe early emotions in other animals too. When my daughter leaves her dog with me while the family goes away for a few days, I see her Grief in the way that she sighs while lying in her basket and even in the way she rouses herself reluctantly when I suggest a walk. I know it is possible to think that humans project these emotions on to other animals, but this research makes a compelling case for emotional capacity at this level being common to all mammals. When in Chapter 5 I examine how we treat the other animals that we eat, I think it may be worth remembering this.

Part three

Here are some case studies to illustrate how the aspects of being human I have described earlier may look in the therapy room.

Case study – the internal critic

'Jack' is not a real person, but a conglomeration of many people I have worked with over the years, both men and women, who experience this kind of punitive inner voice. I don't know whether I see this so much because there are a lot of people out there who experience it or if they are particularly attracted to me, which, I acknowledge, does seem reasonable because of my own process and history.

Jack is slightly overweight. I only notice it because I see the buttons of his formal work shirt bulging. He is well-dressed and self-assured. He tells me he has been experiencing unusually high levels of stress at work and has begun to feel depressed. I ask him what actually happens in his experience that he describes as 'depression'. He says he is unable to go to sleep and feels high levels of anxiety at work. He is reasonably self-possessed when he says this, but I become aware of traces of distress. I slow down and breathe and then I ask him how it feels to be here telling me about this, wondering if there might be some shame being evoked. He looks slightly surprised and then thinks for a moment and says, 'Actually, it's ok. Not as bad as I thought'. I try to reassure him: 'It is odd to be in a room with a stranger and to be talking about these things. . . . What did you expect it to be like?'

'I didn't know. I thought you might have some kind of programme I would follow. . .'.

'I don't work like that, although I know many people who do, and it's useful. But I prefer to work with the relationship between us, how we interact together here – really explore what is possible, and where the limits are. This can be a space to practise different ways of being and see what works. How does that sound?'

Jack looks confused but intrigued. Then he starts to talk about his new boss. They had been colleagues before the new appointment, and my client had also applied unsuccessfully for the job. The culture of the company encouraged competition and fitness. The new boss sometimes talks critically about overweight people saying things like, 'you're too slow if you're fat'. My client thinks he is taking a swipe at him.

'And how do you feel when this happens?' I ask.

His face darkens, he moves uncomfortably in his chair and I can hear it coming. 'I feel worthless, but maybe he's right. . . . After all, I didn't get the job'.

'What was that like for you, not getting the job?' I say.

'I can't get anything right'.

'Can't get anything right'. I repeat it back to him so he can hear the words out loud 'Yet, you appear confident and successful to me, so it doesn't seem likely that can be the whole truth'. He starts to look relieved, but I notice a dangerous edge approaching, where I might find myself giving him the exact same message about getting things wrong as the archaic one he is already carrying to his cost.

'Not that I want to contradict you or criticize in any way. . .'. I add, hoping that this signal that some discrimination is possible, and might be appropriate now, moves us out of danger.

'No' he says, looking like he is feeling a mix of confusion and wonder.

'What's it like to hear me say that?' I ask.

'It's good, actually, gives me a bit of a different perspective. . .'.

I consider asking him whose voice it is he hears saying 'You can't get anything right' when that message goes off in his head, expecting it to be his father's voice, or maybe his mother's or another significant relative or teacher. But we don't have very much time left in this session.

'Would you like to come back another time and explore it a bit more?' I ask.

And, of course, people usually do come back, begin to bring into awareness the negative messages they are carrying that are so deeply embedded that they seem automatic and inevitable. Then they can begin the practice of catching them when they come up and replacing them with something more humane, nuanced and appropriate to the situation. This did not go so well, but that was ok.

Case studies – emotions

Recognizing unexpressed emotion and restoring emotional range is a regular aspect of my work. Here are some examples, and again they are blends of a number of different people and situations.

Alicia – grief, anxiety and perfectionism

Alicia was a busy and generally successful head of department in a secondary school. She usually coped well with the pressures of the role, but in the previous November her father had died, leaving her mother alone and in need of support. As the unmarried daughter in the family, that fell to her. By the following March, she had begun to put on weight. This was unusual for her, and she had noticed that her eating patterns had changed, so she asked to come and have some sessions with me.

I found her gracious, energetic and affable while she explained what had been happening to her. When I asked how she had felt about her father dying, she said she had been upset at first, but was getting over it now. I was suspicious – the way she talked was too controlled – but it was early days and I felt that time was needed in order to build trust. We agreed to meet for six sessions and then review.

Alicia was a 'good' client. She was reliable, prompt and willing to engage with anything I proposed. I was in despair. How was I going to find a way under this facade of bright capability and support her to connect with all the emotion that surely must lie beneath. I talked about her in supervision, acknowledging my own impulse towards being tentative, and my concern that we might have our six sessions and that nothing would have changed for her.

Around session four, she was describing a situation with a junior teacher who had needlessly offended a parent. I could see she was angry, reflected it, and she acknowledged it was the case. 'Did you tell the teacher how angry you were?' I asked her.

She shook her head 'I didn't want to upset her'.

This felt like my opportunity and, very gently, I asked her if she ever didn't want to upset me.

'I never want to upset anyone!' she said, and the tears came then.

We had many more than six sessions. We talked about her grief at her father's death, her anger with the rest of the family for leaving so much to her, her frustration with her mother. She was even able to tell me how annoyed she had been with my early attempts to 'make' her talk when she didn't want to. I saw her anxiety to get things right so that people would like her, the impact of that on her family situation currently. We worked on some alternative strategies and reviewed together the impact of her new and different approach, rejoiced when her brother at last started taking some responsibility for supporting her mother. She lost the weight she had put on too.

Gareth – anger

Gareth was approaching 40 and was living back with his parents for a short time following a divorce. He had no children. I asked him how it was to be back with his family of origin now. He said it was fine – he had his own large bedroom and bathroom and could come and go as he pleased. When he arrived home from work, his mother would be cooking dinner for his father and himself. He said he kept telling her not to bother, but she would insist. He smirked a bit when he said this, and I felt curious about their relationship.

'What does your mother think about the divorce?' I risk, tentatively.

He thinks for a bit. 'I don't think she minds. She never really liked my wife anyway'.

'How was that for you?' I continue.

'It was difficult sometimes. Awkward when we came over – like at Christmas. My mother always insisted that we went there for Christmas lunch. My wife's – ex-wife's – parents lived in Spain, so I don't suppose she thought we had anywhere else to go. . . . She didn't like it though, my ex. . .

'How long had you been married?'

'Five years, but we lived together for eight years before that. We had a big wedding, bridesmaids, church, expensive honeymoon. You know. He shrugs as if all that seems futile now.

'Do you mind my asking . . . what broke you up?'

'Her parents came back from Spain and settled back into the north of England, which is where my wife comes from originally. She went up there to help them settle in and the visits became longer and longer . . . She had to travel a lot for work anyway. . .'. He looks perplexed.

'So even when you were together, you spent a lot of time apart?' I check.

He nods.

'How did you handle it?'

'Oh, I used to go over to mum's, she did my washing and everything. . .'.

'So not much has changed now?' I check out with him.

'Not really. . .'. He looks as though the thought has just occurred to him.

I ask about his childhood and he describes being the precious only son who was given every opportunity in life: university, travel and then a job in the marketing company belonging to a friend of the family.

'How do you get on with your father?' I ask because I feel like something is missing.

He looks puzzled. 'Ok, I suppose. . .'. His voice trails off.

'Does he work?' I find myself interested in this dynamic.

'He's retired now. He used to run his own business – he was away a lot when I was growing up. We had plenty of money because he was so busy, though'.

'It sounds as though you and your mother had to get along with things together a lot of the time', I say. He nods thoughtfully.

My thoughts were moving in the direction of Freud's classic Oedipal triangle and I pulled myself back, wanting to stay with him freshly in the moment, rather than become entangled with preconceived ideas. I was rewarded for my self-discipline when Gareth said:

'I guess I never really got to know him. . .'. (We both know he means his father.)
'Is it too late?' I ask.
'No', he replies simply.

As Gareth finally gets to know his father, he can allow himself to feel anger towards his mother for keeping him so close by, keeping him dependent on her. Our work comes to an end as the sale of the house he had shared with his partner has finalized and he is looking for a flat to move into on his own. He has begun dating again.

Chapter Summary

Each of us has our own way of negotiating our relationship with food. This may work well enough for many people but for others it may bring challenges, sometimes serious, life-threatening ones. We respond to these challenges as whole persons affected physically, mentally, emotionally and relationally. This chapter offered some models for understanding these complex dynamics, always grounded in the assumption that our general state influences what and how we eat (our complex relationship with food) and that our food choices have an effect on our mental health and wellbeing, as well as affecting us physically.

Activities

Please consider the following questions. This may involve thinking about them, meditating on them or making a piece of free-flowing, uncensored writing, similar to those in a personal journal.

3.1 Individual

How would you describe your own relationship with food and how might you connect that to your family of origin?

3.2 With one other person

Think about a negotiation (or consultation) you experienced with a particular person. Do you notice a relational dynamic with this person that reflects the Transactional Analysis ego states? Perhaps you find yourself speaking from a parent ego state. Do you receive a response from the complementary child ego state of the other person? Or is there a cross transaction? Or does something else happen entirely?

3.3 Environment

Where does your food come from? Who chooses it? Who prepares it? How does this affect you and the people around you?

Personal reflection – flying cakes

Written by Piergiulio Poli. Clinical Psychologist, Gestalt Counsellor, Sociologist. Italy.

Maria is 44 years old. Every morning she comes to the mental health community centre where I am doing a placement as a trainee counsellor. She lives in the council houses a block away from the centre, which is in Turin, northern Italy. Maria lives with her mother, a southern Italian 'mama', now in her 70s. Everly morning Maria walks the ten minutes from home to here and when she arrives, she is exhausted. She now weighs around 130 kg, which is more than 20 stone, and that is a lot of weight to carry around even for a short walk. When Maria comes through the door, she is red in the face and panting heavily. She makes for the large sofa where she can finally sit and have a rest. The medication the psychiatrists have been prescribing for her for the last 10 years tends to make her a bit dull and terribly hungry. Eating is her trade-off with the people in her world and the price she has to pay to find some acceptance.

Her mother loves her and possibly hates her too. She feeds Maria way too much. Maria doesn't know how to say no to some fettuccine, especially if it is cooked by mama. In fact, she doesn't know how to say no to anything. Dad has never been there, he left Maria and her mother many, many years ago. Since that time, they have lived together, often sleeping in the same bed, and never leaving the vast social housing complex on the outskirts of the city. In the community centre Maria, for the first time in her life, learns to cook for herself, and how to choose healthy food. Mama sometimes comes in when Maria and the other patients cook with the help of a nutritionist. This is something new for her too. The therapeutic work Maria and I do together is focussed on the possibility of her being able to say no.

One day there is a party in the community centre. The table is full of cakes the patients have baked, and there are soft drinks and some singing – we are having a good time. Maria is in a good mood. She comes over to me and I joke with her saying, 'There are cakes flying all around us today!'. She looks at me with bright eyes, truly happy. She says 'Yes, and I do not have to eat all of them!'.

Food note

Who'll be eating my porridge?

I buy my oats from the organic stores, levering them cautiously out of the hopper into a stout paper bag and when I get home, cascading them into a big glass storage jar, where they sit under their measuring cup until I scoop them into a saucepan early in the morning. I like to shake my panful flat, sprinkle it with sea salt and leave it to soak for a while in a minimal amount of cold water.

Porridge is personal. Like the three bears in the story, we each have our individual preferences. I like mine almost the consistency of pale hummus, so I stir from the moment I switch the gas on to the lowest light possible and keep going until the contents become unctuous. At a country house I stayed in while taking a food writing course, the chef preserved the integrity of each little oat and served her porridge like jewels suspended in milkiness. I've also hacked wedges from a pan that had been sitting all night at the bottom of an Aga while staying in a spiritual community, the porridge tasting smoky and toasty.

Fruit and a spoon of yoghurt, maybe with a couple of walnuts crumbled on top, maple syrup or, for a special treat at Christmas, double cream and demerara sugar are my favourite toppings.

Piling the cooked porridge out into a dish means running the risk of leaving a lot of breakfast around the sides of the pan. I use a scraper to make sure I don't miss out on any of my portion. I've heard 'food people' call pan-scrapers 'child-cheaters' because using them means that there is no cake-mixture left in the bowl for a child (or anyone) to smear off with their fingers and send up into their mouths. I imagine Goldilocks felt cheated when the three bears came back and she had to run off into the forest. Perhaps there was porridge, as she liked it, for her own breakfast when she arrived safely home.

References

Berne, E. (1988) *What do you say after you say hello*. London: Corgi Books.
Carter, R. (2019) *The brain book*. London: Dorling Kindersley.
Damasio, A. (2000) *The feeling of what happens*. London: Vintage.
Geary, A. (2001) *The food and mood handbook*. London: Thorsons.
Jacka, F. (2019) *Brainchanger*. Great Britain: Yellow Kite.
Korn, L. (2016) *Nutrition essentials for mental health*. New York: Norton.
Mayer, E. (2016) *The mind-gut connection*. New York: Harper Collins.
Melchert, N. (2014) *The great conversation*. New York: Oxford University Press.
Panksepp, J. and Biven, L. (2012) *The archaeology of mind*. New York: Norton.
Procyk, A. (2018) *Nutritional treatments to improve mental health disorders*. Eau Claire, WI: Pesi Publishing and Media.

4 Wholeness, balance and regulation

Needs and Gestalt

Introduction

The chapter begins with an exploration of needs, in relation to food and to life in general. Human beings have a whole range of different needs, many of which can only be addressed by reaching out to other people or to the physical, social or other aspects of the arena in which our lives unfold.

The relationship between a person and their environment is further examined by introducing some ideas from Gestalt. This is a whole-person approach offering a theory of perception, a model for psychotherapy and a philosophy of living. Fundamental to its thinking is the relationship between self and other, the inevitability of interconnectedness between an individual and the rest of the world, and the dynamics of our relational fields.

The exploration hopes to offer fresh insights about the fundamental connection between our experience of food and our experience of life in general, contributing to the outline of mental (and physical) health that I am attempting to distil. It may also suggest new possibilities for one-to-one work with clients, groups and the wider field.

Chapter structure

Part One surveys the range of different needs associated with being human.

Part Two describes the relational process that takes place as an individual interacts with what is available in the environment in order to meet these essential needs. The Gestalt approach is used as a lens for understanding this dynamic.

Part Three explores the process more deeply, focusing on how we recognize the needs that are most significant in the moment. In this way, we can avoid the possible tendency to distract ourselves into old patterns of behaviour. These may cause us to attempt to meet different needs, so failing to satisfy the authentic appetite. Various possibilities are presented through case studies of clients in psychotherapy. (This section is written by Dr Di Hodgson.)

DOI: 10.4324/9781003172161-5

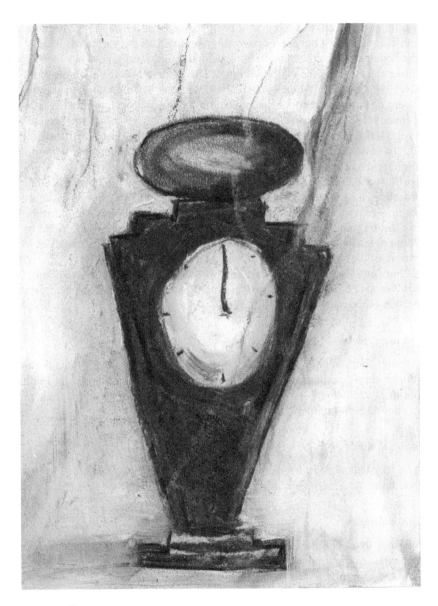

Weighing it all up

Part one

Needs – 'the need organizes the field' Lewin 1926

Being human and alive is a dynamic, complex process. How do we organize all the different facets of our selves in relationship with all the various aspects of our environment so as to create a satisfying outcome for us as individuals, for the people around us and for the wider field too? The aforementioned quote from Lewin (1926/1999, quoted in Wollants, 2012, p. 9) suggests that directing our attention to fulfilling our own current dominant need offers one approach to the resolution of that endeavour. This may seem self-centred at first but, as well as the need organizing the field, it is also true that 'the field influences the need' (Wollants, 2012, p. 9). By answering our own needs, we can also be responding in relation to our environment and influencing others.

To illustrate this by a focus on food, think about how a clock indicating the approach of lunchtime in a work day, which is an outside stimulus, can arouse appetite as much as an empty feeling in the stomach, which is an internal stimulus, does. The fragrance of coffee, the sweet wholesomeness of baking bread or the perfume of garlic and spice can all result in a sensation of the taste buds at whatever time of day. Yet food is more than just a physical need.

As humans, we have needs that are physical, emotional, intellectual and relational. We also have needs that we might call spiritual. Here are some examples (the list is not exhaustive):

Physical needs

Air, water, food, shelter, movement, exertion, relaxation, sleep, touch, instinct, health, sickness, healing, sex, crying, screaming, sighing, laughing, 'gut-feelings' (intuition?), attunement – somehow tuning into the same energetic frequency with others and the environment, death.

Emotional needs

Safety, jeopardy (but not too much), security, consistency, novelty, belonging, individuality, love, hate, joy, anger, despair, fear, jealousy, envy, pleasure, etc.

Relational needs

Belonging, love, care, approval, appreciation, challenge, sex, romance, shared humanity, identification with the natural world, pets, associations, commerce, businesses, religions, shared hobbies, interests and causes.

Intellectual needs

Ideas, understanding, learning, synthesizing, analysing, focusing, integrating, information-gathering, creativity, intelligence, decision making, etc.

Spiritual needs

Beauty, awe, transcendency, meaning, universality, stories, sacredness, images, rituals, music, art, poetry, delight, religion, the transcendent or numinous.

Food is connected with the satisfaction of all the different kinds of needs I have identified. It provides us with the physical sustenance we need to fuel our bodies, plus the satisfaction of smell, taste, consistency and feel – feeling in the mouth and stomach, but also of the hand: an apple, a sandwich, a chocolate biscuit or a morsel of cheese; the satisfaction of the action of hand to mouth.

The physical sensation of being 'well-fed' brings the emotional satisfaction of pleasure, security, consistency and variety. Mealtimes connect us with families and friends, the natural world that provides so much variety and abundance (hopefully) and the farmers, shopkeepers or chefs that contributed to its arrival on our tables. The type of food we eat and the way we prepare and serve it are fundamental markers of a shared culture. Being invited to participate in someone else's food culture has a significance beyond the excitement of unfamiliar ingredients, combinations and tastes; it also offers possibilities for increased inclusivity and understanding. Our intellects are fed by knowledge of nutrient values, production methods or sources; understanding how food affects our bodies and the world in which we live resources us. Finally, ritual meals are part of the practice of worship in many religions. At the same time, meals can be secular rituals that bring meaning, sacredness, delight and beauty to our everyday experience.

Needs are a fundamental facet of our interconnectedness with the world around us. We reach out into our environment and are met with some kind of more or less satisfactory response. We have a whole vocabulary for describing the nuances of these interactions and the various levels of intensity involved. Acting on a whim by popping a piece of chocolate into my mouth is much less significant for me than making a passionate commitment to creating a meaningful life. That chocolate may provide me with a rapturous moment, but it is temporary and soon forgotten. Investing time and energy in anything that is meaningful for me, like building family relationships or, indeed, writing a book, is longer term, requires more sustained effort and, eventually, delivers a more satisfying outcome.

The significance and urgency of the investment of our time and energy influence the level of satisfaction we achieve from the potential consequences. What we choose to invest our time and energy into is a powerful expression of our unique selves. In real life, we need to be involved in the whole range of possible interactions, from a tiny edible treat to significant life achievements. These various aspects of experience happen sometimes simultaneously and sometimes consecutively. I can eat chocolate while I work on my computer, but I can't be available to really meet with a client unless I give the situation my full attention. The different facets of our lives become embedded around one another and the reverberations of the ongoing elements over time shape the development of our lives (Wheeler, 1998).

We also have words to describe the emotional quality of our reaching into the world. Hunger is the prerequisite for satisfaction, whether the object is food or any other need. Desire is more piquant than necessity and adds richness to our experience of being alive. We may venture into the world with a powerful intention to make something happen; alternatively, we may observe what is being offered to us by the environment and accept that. Reaching out with our whims, passions, desires, interest and attention has a responding impact on the parts of the environment with which we connect: the chocolate is assimilated into my body, my family members grow and thrive, people eventually read the book and are (hopefully) interested in the ideas and take them forward into their own lives.

In his book 'Seven Brief Lessons on Physics' (2016), Carlo Rovelli describes the behaviour of electrons in Quantum Theory:

> They only exist when someone or something watches them, or better, when they are interacting with something else. They materialize in a place, with a calculable probability, when colliding with something else. . . . In quantum mechanics no object has a definite position, except when colliding headlong with something else.
>
> (p. 15)

Maybe there is a truth in this for human beings in the 'big' world too. It is certainly my experience that I become myself in my interactions with other people, things and ideas. I have also noticed that by giving attention to something I make it grow, whether it is the snowdrops growing in my garden, the people with whom I work or my ideas about how to live a fulfilling life.

Gestalt

The ability to regulate our relationships with food (and life in general) can be supported by methodologies that are holistic, relational and grounded in context. Gestalt is the approach that formed the basis of my training as a psychotherapist and it has informed my understanding of how humans regulate interactions with the people and things around us. Its theory and practice are grounded in that relationship with 'other' in which each individual constantly participates. Here is something of its history.

Historical background

The founders of Gestalt were Fritz and Laura Perls and Paul Goodman (Humphrey, 1986 in Clarkson and Mackewn, 1993). Fritz was born in a Jewish neighbourhood of Berlin in 1893. During the First World War, he worked in the trenches as a medical officer and afterwards qualified as a neuropsychiatrist setting up a practice in Berlin, where he mixed with philosophers, artists and dancers, becoming part of the between-the-wars 'Bohemian community' (Clarkson and Mackewn, 1993, p. 5) that has since become legendary. In 1928, he qualified as a Freudian psychoanalyst.

Fritz and Laura married in 1929, although they had been in relationship for some years before that. Her background was as an academic studying gestalt psychology and she was also familiar with existentialism and phenomenology (p. 11). After some time in Holland, they moved to South Africa, where they had two children. After the Second World War, in 1946, the family moved to New York (Clarkson and Mackewn, 1993).

Before he became involved with Gestalt, Goodman had been a poet and playwright and was interested in social issues and education. He met with Fritz and Laura Perls when they came to Manhattan from Europe (Stoehr, 1994). I imagine him as one of the cool, clever, innovative New Yorkers of the mid-twentieth century. Together, these three developed a new approach to psychotherapeutic work.

Fritz and Laura both trained and practised as psychoanalysts and continued to call themselves analysts for much of their careers. The traditional analytic approach, after Freud (1905), was for patients to be lying on a couch with the analyst seated behind them, out of sight. Developments in the field at that time were changing that arrangement to one in which patient and analyst both sat in chairs and faced one another, and Fritz and Laura preferred this method. They were influenced by the work of Wilhelm Reich, which was centred on the body, so the new approach they developed gave primacy to the body, to awareness of what was currently being experienced and to describing what could be observed in the present moment (Perls, 1992b). This method of describing actual experience was different from the usual analytic practice of making interpretations based on theory. Gestalt developed into an approach in which intense and lively contact between therapist and client (and between participants in training workshops, of which there were many) became the primary aim. The authentic expression of the individual was prized, reflecting the environment of freedom and self-expression that was happening in the west in the 1960s. Since then, again reflecting how society in general has been developing, Gestalt has become more professional and the balance has adjusted between recognizing the wants and needs of the individual, and acknowledging those of the environment, whether that is in the context of therapy, or in families, neighbourhoods and society. The foundational text of the approach is called 'Gestalt Therapy: Excitement and Growth in the Human Personality', which was originally published in 1951. The edition I use is a later one (Perls, Hefferline and Goodman, 1992).

Ego, hunger and aggression

Before that, in 1947, Perls' first published work was called 'Ego Hunger and Aggression', which was written during the time his own children were young. In it, he acknowledged the parallels between how we take in and process life, and how we take in and process food, and established this understanding as a central aspect of his approach. He observed the series of sucking, biting and chewing through which infants progress and related them to adult life. Without teeth, we can only take in specialized liquid forms of nourishment, crucially breast milk or an equivalent formula. While the nature and means of gaining nourishment are limited, and the provision entirely dependent on another person, it seems to me that there is nothing half-hearted about how it is received. Even tiny newborns suck ferociously, as anyone whose finger has been grabbed by a baby's ever-vigilant mouth can confirm. While appetite can be urgent, the mechanisms that enable us to recognize when we've had enough are already in place – a full tummy and the satisfaction in lips, mouth and jaw that follows meaningful activity, plus the comfort of being warmly held and the sensation of the skin of hand or breast. Anything that cannot be assimilated returns fairly soon via the way it came in.

With the development of the front teeth, we are able to bite off pieces from a larger, solid item: banana, bread, a carrot or a cracker, which is usually grasped in the child's hand. At this point, we can consider a variety of possibilities on a plate and reach out to take what suits us best at the time. After practice, we can use our teeth, tongue and jaw to convert the small lump we have bitten off into something soft enough to slide easily down the throat. Or else we can spit it out voluntarily – the beginning of the 'no' that characterizes a 2-year-old. By the time our back teeth arrive, we have even more selectivity because we can name what we want and even open the cupboard door of where it is kept. We can tear and chew, digest and fully assimilate what we take in – eating and living as a way of aggressing into the environment and creating satisfaction.

For a baby, it is obvious that the exchange with the 'environment' – other people who earn the money to buy, and go shopping for, the formula or food, lift the baby into the high-chair, pass the sippy-cup and so on – is essential to the point where it is undisputedly necessary for survival. The impact of caring for a baby is equally powerful, although usually more life-changing than life-threatening. As we become adults, earn our own money and provide our own meals, the exchange with the environment becomes less evident, but it still exists. Perls insists that 'No organism is self-sufficient. It requires the world for the gratification of its needs' (1992a, p. 34).

As adults, we make decisions about the food we obtain, where it comes from and who cooks what we eat that impact on family relationships, the hospitality and retail industries and society in general. The growers or producers, the vans or lorries that deliver the commodities, and the shops and supermarkets in our neighbourhoods are necessary for the comfort of all of us. When food supply becomes uncertain, as it did in the 2020 Covid epidemic, the significance of our inter-relatedness comes into focus again. Our 'environment': staff in restaurants and takeaway outlets, shop-workers, delivery-drivers, farmers, supermarket bosses and politicians all have an effect on us, and we both by our choices of where and how to spend our money, and where we cast our votes have an effect on them.

For those of us who work with other people in formal, contracted roles, it is likely that we notice that not only do we have an effect on our clients, but they have an effect on us too. Being aware of the effect we have on each other and contextualizing that particular exchange within the wider environment in which it is situated can help us become more effective and not only when we are directly concerned with food and mental health.

It can be revealing to parallel the relational styles we observe happening between ourselves and the people with whom we work with the process of eating and digestion. Do I expect that my suggestions or insights will be swallowed whole? Do I notice when my client (or I) hold something in our metaphorical mouths, ready to spit it out later? What happens when a client 'spits out' (or vomits) what I have to offer? What happens when it sticks in the gut and can't be assimilated? None of the ways in which we integrate or reject 'other' is necessarily right or wrong; it depends on the present circumstances, and those change constantly. This is why being able to observe and make sense of whatever happens is a valuable professional skill. Using eating as a metaphor can be an accessible way to think and talk about our experience. 'Science can speak of a balanced diet only if all the different kinds of hunger instincts are satisfied' (Perls, Hefferline and Goodman, 1992, p. 3).

Experience and interconnectedness

Human beings have a unique way of experiencing existence, influenced by the development of a mind that enables us to have a sense of being a unique self, separate from but connected with everything that exists outside ourselves. What I call environment or world is what we experience as other than our unique self. This includes other people, of course, but also non-human beings like pets, trees, berries and woodlice and the earth, sky and air, as well as houses and roads, shops and food, laptops and books, and the weather.

Contact boundary

The hypothetical 'join' between person and world in Gestalt is called the 'contact boundary', which Merleau-Ponty (1964/1968, p. 235; in Wollants, 2012, p. 53) defines as a 'surface of separation between me and the other, which is also the place of our union'. I imagine it like a sinuous continuum, responsive to the flow of connectedness that is sometimes initiated by the person and other times required by the world. 'The behaviour of the person is as much initiated by forces arising from the experienced requirements of the situation as it is by the egocentric forces within the person' (Wollants, 2012, p. 55).

Contact boundary is a metaphor. Of course, it is not really a line, although to help understanding it may be thought of as one. The constraints of language invite the reduction of a dynamic, complex and vivid process into a 'thing' that can be understood, mastered and used. While my intention is always to avoid any diminishment of this kind if I can, I understand that human beings like metaphor, we respond to it and it helps us learn in a way that is different from the rational linearity of thought. Psychoanalyst and story specialist Bruno Bettelheim (1976, p. 31) identified that 'a child's unconscious processes can become clarified for him only through images which speak directly to his unconscious'. This is the language of analysis, but it does recognize that the irrational and imaginative aspects of being human are significant and have their own contribution to make to our understanding of the world we inhabit and, I believe, not only when we are children. I offer metaphors and illustrations in that spirit.

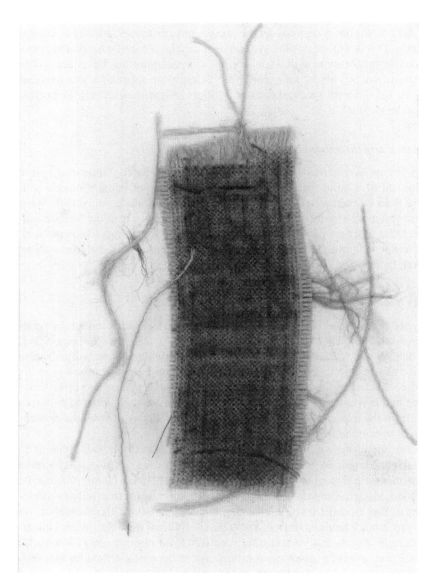

Restoring threads of energy emerge from a seam of contact

As relationships with food are the focus of this book, I will begin discussing the application of the metaphor of the contact boundary by giving an example of an interaction that is based around eating. On one side of the imaginary seam that is the contact boundary I am present in my body, mind, emotions and other parts of my self. My different facets may be in general agreement with one another, or they may be in conflict. I may be aware of how peaceful or conflicted they are, but I may well not be aware of everything I am experiencing. Deep in the cells and tissues of my body lie the memories of my past experiences in relation to food, many of them dating from before I could speak, so not easily accessible to my thought process. I also have a variety of different needs that may potentially be clamouring for my attention in the present moment.

Food is on the other side of the imaginary contact boundary. Potentially all the food in the world, although there are constraints like ease of availability, cost and personal taste that restrict the choice quite considerably. The process of choosing what to eat for supper this evening, even if only from just everything easily available to me, could still be bewildering. In practice, I have learned habits that allow me to put a meal together without having to re-invent my whole capacity for decision making every time. I usually choose something from the food items I have bought previously and so are available in my house (see the Food Note following for more detail). Other people may drop into the supermarket on the way home and pick up something from the shelves that seems attractive to them in the moment. Still others might pick up their phones and choose to have a fully prepared meal delivered to them, wherever they are. The interaction between an individual and something compellingly interesting in the environment creates a thread of energy (a bit like those in the illustration) that involves each of the 'sides' in some kind of active involvement leading to a resolution that changes both, sometimes subtly, occasionally very significantly.

Whatever the route, the food arrives on my plate and I lift my fork to spear my first mouthful. Usually, I am guided by the sight and smell of the food, and the signals in my mouth and stomach that leap forward in response to the present encounter. Much less evident to me by that time are the resolutions I may have made about losing a few pounds or avoiding refined carbohydrates. Other people have different responses. For some, the danger of putting on weight may cause anxiety or revulsion. Others may desensitize and shovel the food down as fast as possible, having become accustomed to situations in the past where there are a lot of competing hungry mouths or an actual shortage of food. Then comes the dilemma of when to stop. This is always difficult for me because I was encouraged as a child to clear my plate, not to let things go to waste. I still dislike wasting food, but I have developed the capacity to make better decisions than the old strategy of over-filling myself. One of the ways I have developed for dealing with this dilemma is to serve myself a small portion, but have more of whatever it is available, so I know it is there if I want it. Usually, I don't want it, and I have some delicious leftovers available for another meal.

Things other than food are also present on the other side of the contact boundary, like the conditions in my current physical environment. For example, I may choose to go out for a walk but then it begins to rain. I may notice the sky darkening, and then sense the first drops falling on my hair. I am likely to experience an emotional response, maybe of annoyance, or disappointment or even pleasure, depending on my general mood and the circumstances in which I am taking the walk. Then I have a choice to make; either get wet, find some shelter or put up the umbrella I had the forethought to bring with me. . . . I decide how I will respond and take some action. Then I encounter the consequences of my choice, which may be comfortable and satisfying, like walking with my umbrella in the rain, in which case I will continue doing that until I feel uncomfortable again. Maybe my shoe begins to let in water, which means I am experiencing a different discomfort now, so the cycle – body sensation, feelings, decisions, action – reconstitutes, resulting in different consequences which I experience as either more or less satisfying.

Continuity of connectedness

Let's return to the contact boundary. If I try to visualize it diagrammatically, I see a line that begins (hypothetically) at my birth. The point at which it ends is now. Yet, in reality, it does not end, because the next 'now' arrives, and I anticipate that the association between me and my world, illustrated by the imaginary line depicting the contact boundary between us, will continue for some time, until I eventually die. While past and future are present implicitly, my involvement is with a sequence of successive 'nows', which I experience as being my existence (Sartre, 1984). 'Now' can be powerful and exciting. It is where the possibility lies for creating an interesting and meaningful life. 'Now' can also stressful and intimidating because things may just not come to pass as well as I had intended.

Experiment – an imaginary 'other'

*I decide to use this section of writing as a lens for observing how my own internal process unfolds in my current experience of 'now'. I continue to type in good faith. Ten seconds ago, I paused and decided to change the font to italics, in an effort to make what I am doing clearer to the reader. If you **are** reading this, it means that the passage has survived several edits and made it to the final version. Is what I am trying to demonstrate actually clearer for you because I have italicized this passage? Does describing my own experience and thought process clarify the theory I am trying to explain?*

(This experiment has actually also turned out to be a demonstration of how, even though you are not physically present to me now, I still have a concept of you, and I am making an effort to connect with you in a way that is interesting and meaningful. This capacity to imagine scenarios that have not taken place yet or, indeed, may never happen is unique to us as humans. Our imaginations allow us to consider 'what if?' scenarios which are the basis of creativity, and

also contribute to our being able to have empathy with others. We can imagine how others are feeling even if we are not experiencing the same feelings currently ourselves, and even if we have never actually felt them and never will).

Learning from experience

In writing, when things do not turn out as I had hoped, I can always delete and try again. Can I do that in other aspects of my life? Well, my subjective response is that sometimes I can, and other times I can't. Take my example of walking in the rain in the previous section. What if I had wanted to continue with my walk but had forgotten to bring my umbrella, and also felt reluctant to get wet because I was meeting a friend, so didn't want to sit dripping in the coffee shop? Well, I would make some choice based on my current needs and priorities to resolve that situation: probably either put up with getting wet or else go home for my umbrella and text my friend to say I will be late. This is what is called a 'creative adjustment'. But I would be likelier to remember to bring my umbrella another time.

Each moment offers an opportunity for 'excitement and growth' (to quote part of the subtitle of 'Gestalt Therapy'). Yet the actual outcome of our engagement with the moment may feel drab and bleak, or more stressful than we can assimilate, and this is part of living too. Understanding more about the process means we have greater choice in the way we respond and allows us an increased possibility for more sparkling (or reassuring) outcomes down the line.

Figure and ground

The German word 'gestalt', for which there is no direct English equivalent, describes a complete picture. It is a term used also by visual artists, which refers to perception: the way our senses (in this case the visual) deliver our current experience of our world to us in time. In 'Ways of Seeing' (Berger, 1972, p. 9), art critic John Berger observes,

> Soon after we can see, we are aware that we can also be seen. The eye of the other combines with our own eye to make it fully credible that we are part of the visible world. . . . The reciprocal nature of vision is more fundamental than that of the spoken word.

For both artists and Gestaltists sensing is a relational experience.

A 'gestalt' is an element of experience that feels whole and has meaning. The gestalt is a complete picture because it is organized into a foreground or 'figure' and a background. In art, this is called 'composition'. Berger writes 'The compositional unity of a painting contributes fundamentally to the power of its image' and goes on to explain how composition can contribute to depicting the 'unchanging human condition' (p. 13). At the hypothetical contact boundary or, to put it more accurately, in life, the current situation or our experience of here-and-now is foreground and what has come before and what may happen afterwards constellate into a multi-faceted background (Wheeler, 1998). Just like with the landscape behind the smiling face of Monalisa, both figure and ground are visible, but meaning derives from the dynamic between them.

Individual and environment

Experience at the contact boundary can be relatively tranquil, with me and my environment moving along together harmoniously, having nothing to disturb our process through time. Then often, and inevitably, something disturbs our equilibrium. The reason for the imbalance may belong more to me, some indistinct unease that begins to emerge, or it may belong more to the environment, the doorbell rings. In the latter case, the ringing doorbell demands a response. My body 'jumps' at the sudden, intrusive sound, I become aware of an increasing energy in my chest that I quickly identify as anticipation, 'It's my parcel!', I realize. I get to my feet and rush to the door, turn the latch and open to the sight of a delivery man holding out a brown box. Automatically, my hand reaches to take the box from him, and I smile and say 'thank-you'. He turns away as I close the door and bring the parcel inside. I open it and take out the contents. Yes, it is the book I've been waiting for. . . . I notice a lightness in my chest that I recognize as pleasure, confirmed by the sensation that the corners of my mouth are lifting. Then I put the book aside, turn back to my laptop and continue with the piece of work I had been doing.

Some time later, my eyes lift from the screen, I draw in a noticeably larger breath and shift about on my seat. What has disturbed me? I start to speculate in an unfocused way . . . Ah! A hollow sensation in my stomach emerges into my awareness. I look at the clock. Lunchtime. I joyfully abandon my laptop and reach for the kettle.

Whether the disequilibrium is situated more with me, or with my environment, both 'sides' of the contact boundary adjust to the new situation and are changed by it. The delivery man gets back into his van and searches for his next address. I have the book I need, and I can look at it later in the afternoon. After I've eaten my lunch. I rinse out the empty milk carton and put it in the recycling. This choice will have an impact on the environment too, down the line.

The future is not really 'down the line' of the contact boundary, yet it is helpful to have a metaphorical way to connect now with a potential future, particularly because we understand that our experience now influences what will happen later. This quote from Buddha (in Kumar, 2017, p. 65) is a well-known teaching that seems to underline how choices in the moment have a potential long-term impact:

> The thought manifests as the word;
> The word manifests as the deed;
> The deed develops the habit;
> And habit hardens into character.

The unfolding of experience at my contact boundary may be a path towards my future, but it is not a fixed path: there is no inevitability about the kind of person I am becoming, or the world I am contributing towards creating. The way is hacked out through struggle and pain, excitement and pleasure. The 'direction' it takes reflects all those past decisions. . .

Elements of experience (gestalts)

We are beginning to recognize elements of experience that start with a response to a disturbance, and that gradually become more fully understood and identifiable, until there is some kind of exchange between person and environment, which is the resolution of that particular situation. Then there is a process of assimilation and hopefully of integration and meaning making (the previous discussion of how we encounter food by sucking, biting and chewing offers some suggestions for the kind of outcomes that might be possible). At the close of an experiential episode, some sort of balance point is achieved and then, when the time is right, another element of experience can emerge. Where does it come from? Out of the interaction between person and world, in the context of the momentary shared situation. Some imbalance (or disequilibrium) is experienced, identified by Wollants (p. 55) as potentially being initiated by either the person or the environment. In the previous example, the rain would be an environmentally initiated factor. An example of a factor initiated by the person might be that, while I am enjoying my walk, I suddenly remember that I may have forgotten to turn off the gas after I finished making toast earlier (something I do quite often) and I rush home to check. My focus has changed, and the former tranquillity of my environment is disrupted by someone running along with an umbrella.

Focus on a person-initiated element of experience

There is a kind of harmony, or unity, between person and world until an imbalance occurs, and the mutual quest for resolution is begun. While both individual and environment are involved and affected, our main concern here is the response of the individual person. As human beings, this involvement is familiar to each of us, even if we haven't imagined it to be that way until now. It is how we experience our existence and we have evolved in relation to it. Indeed, we keep on evolving in relation to it as we live our lives. The ease, grace and effectiveness of our engagement in the process of its unfolding influences whether we feel we have a good life or not.

In order for the exchange between human and world to happen, differentiation needs to be heightened. I need to sink my teeth into the apple, tear off the flesh, spit out the pips, grind the flesh to pulp and swallow it down. Or I need to grapple with an idea (as maybe you are now), rigorously check it out, tear it apart to discover inconsistencies or unpalatable parts, think about it, notice my feelings of fascination or frustration (or both), smugness or inadequacy, maybe try it out tentatively to discover what happens.

The process is similar with another person, although there are two subjectivities involved then: me and you. In the ordinary way, we often connect with one another one person at a time, even though there might be others present. For example, I may chat to my grandson about his new toy fire truck, while other family members are busy making dinner. In a shop or café, my interaction is generally with one other person at a time, as I make my purchase. There are, of course, situations where the exchange is with more than one person. Team meetings, for example, or meals with friends, and these bring additional complexity.

Whether these exchanges are with groups or one-to-one, there will be different levels of investment required of us in order to achieve the resolution we need or want. Perhaps, German philosopher Martin Büber expresses this most profoundly in his theory of 'I-Thou' (Büber, 1958/1984). He contrasts a mutual, receptive, immediate exchange that is redolent with shared humanity called 'I-Thou', with a functional, perfunctory transaction called 'I-It'. Both are necessary. The first is required for building close, meaningful, fulfilling relationships. The second is fine if the need is just for a cup of coffee.

In order to meet with you in an 'I-Thou' way I need to become as fully myself as I can, while you become similarly fully yourself. This may sound counterintuitive: surely, we look for relationship in closeness? While some real connectedness is certainly necessary, sameness is not. The most meaningful interactions take place when each participant can differentiate, embody the self-other dynamic and enjoy a lively, creative exchange. This kind of encounter leaves both parties different from who they were before.

Cycles of experience

When the equilibrium between me and my environment tips out of balance, the process of resolution requires me to engage in the situation with as many of my faculties as I can. You will notice from the examples that body sensation is often the first indication that a fresh gestalt (unit of experience) has begun: I feel rain on my hair, I notice gnawings in my stomach, I hear the doorbell ring. . . . Some emotional reaction comes into my awareness: dismay that it has begun to rain, pleasure that it's lunchtime, surprise. . . . I begin to consider possibilities: is the rain heavy enough for me to need to get my umbrella out? Shall I go home? Is it salad for lunch today, or do I really need a sandwich? Who is at the door? Is it the book I ordered? I decide how I will respond and take action. The situation resolves in the best way it can with the resources and constraints that are available. I walk on under my umbrella and meet my friend at the coffee shop, I eat lunch, I answer the door. . . . Then I have a reaction to my choice: I'm glad I met my friend, I wish I'd chosen the salad, I'm pleased the book arrived. . . . Eventually, equilibrium is restored. Of course, this is a simplification, but you can check it out for yourself any time – after all, this is how we experience our lives moment by moment. . .

What need is being met?

Written by Dr Di Hodgson, a Gestalt psychotherapist, supervisor and trainer with 30 years' experience, Director of Studies for the MSc in Gestalt psychotherapy at the Metanoia Institute UK, member of the editorial team of the British Gestalt Journal, a regular facilitator of workshops at National and International Conferences, and a visiting trainer and external examiner at several institutes across Europe.

As described earlier, in Gestalt theory, food has been a metaphor from the outset. Perls, Hefferline and Goodman (abbreviated to PHG subsequently) include it in their original developmental theory (1977 [1951]), and it continues to be part of our clinical thinking in reality and in metaphor, not least in terms of boundaries and how these are negotiated in relationship. Central to Gestalt theory are what were originally known as 'interruptions to contact', which then resulted in 'contact boundary disturbances'. These ideas have been developed over time and are now understood as 'moderations' (Wheeler, 1991) or 'modifications' (Yontef, 1993), where no position is intrinsically positive or negative, but rather that their usefulness depends on the situation and our capacity to move flexibility along a continuum. In addition, the Cycle of Experience, also outlined earlier, describes a rhythm whereby we become aware of our needs, mobilize to meet them and, if all goes well, experience satisfaction. In therapy, we often see how there are problems at any stage in the cycle. We often find that a client may not know what their needs are, which may be a disturbance between sensation and awareness, or they may mobilize towards meeting the 'wrong' need or suppress the need. Often, in these situations, the need is mis-labelled and therefore the 'wrong' need is attended to, most obviously, for example, in addictive behaviours. In these cases, the person knows that they need something; however, they typically mobilize towards something that provides temporary satisfaction or that avoids the feelings that are associated with acknowledging the need, and so the need remains unmet. This process of interruption or distortion becomes a cycle or fixed Gestalt (ibid) in itself.

PHG's developmental theory includes the important act of chewing, as distinct from swallowing whole or spitting out. Not so literally, this process can be seen in our ability to chew over ideas, suggestions, advice, etc., rather than swallowing or dismissing someone else's perspective.

This 'swallowing whole' commonly applies to concepts, standards of behaviour and facts, as well as to food, and can be understood in terms of what PHG refer to as 'introjecting' (Perls, Hefferline and Goodman, 1977 [1951], p. 62). These 'introjects' (ibid: 230) are most commonly understood as the 'shoulds' of living. Some 'shoulds' require no chewing over and come under the category of common sense. Most, however, are undigested or indigestible when not chewed sufficiently. Often, they are out of our awareness and act as implicit as well as explicit rules for living. This concept of chewing means that not only are we concerned with whether we let something in, but how we do so.

It is interesting how often relationships with food, in reality and as a metaphor, come up in therapy even when there is no significant eating disorder or disordered eating. Food and need are often intrinsically connected.

The following examples illustrate the vivid, vital and visceral role which food plays.

Case study – Chris

One client Chris (pseudonym) has been in therapy with me for several years. He suffered various developmental traumas as a young child. Consequently, other than playing sport as a teenager (in ways which were often destructive to himself and others), he learned to live mainly in his head, prioritizing his intellect over his body and his felt experience. He literally chose food from a habitual and bland diet.

A recurrent theme in his friendships was his pattern of giving and receiving and how he was far more comfortable giving than receiving in all aspects of his life, including presents, help, time, support, knowledge, etc. Some of Chris's habitual behaviours could be seen through the lens of the Cycle, for example, his giving to, and doing for, others could be understood as him disowning and projecting his needs for attention and care onto others, or in Crocker's terms, proflection (1981) where someone does to, or for, others what they want or need for themselves. Many of his relationships were structured around his being a caretaker, often, again, to his own detriment.

Chris has recently had his first successful, albeit short, relationship with a partner. During lockdown, he has learned to bake cakes, to some extent fuelled by his newfound interest in making his environment more homely, which includes cooking for himself, a skill which he developed whilst being in this recent relationship. During lockdown, he decided to bake and deliver cakes to local friends and their children. At first, this was a familiar theme of his providing for others. It was several weeks before he recalled how his aunts would make cakes for him when he was a small boy. He often struggles to recall positive memories from his childhood, which was otherwise and often described as lonely, brutal, exposing, to name a few. He infamously has years of birthday presents, unopened, on top of his wardrobes. This recent recollection of being baked cakes by his aunts is one profound memory of what and how he could receive, and now he recalls it as a clear expression of love.

This taking in and keeping out can be seen through a lens of 'healthy permeability', that is the capacity to decide for ourselves what is potentially good and nourishing and what is potentially harmful or toxic. I have often used the metaphor of a colander to represent a boundary with clients. Often, they arrive in therapy with the colander working the wrong way round, which means that anything positive from the environment effectively bounces off the metal, whilst what is potentially or actually harmful passes through the holes. To some extent this can be explained by Yontef (1993), who states that positives are like Teflon and negatives like Velcro (which will come as no surprise to many of us!). In the case of my client Chris, I would sometimes experience a very powerful, almost toddler-like resistance to anything positive: a profound unwillingness to improve his situation, a feeling of spitting out. There was an almost ironic resistance to understanding and responding to his needs. He seemed to be both starving and tight-lipped at the same time. One might say that one of the tasks of therapy was to understand and experiment with this colander effect, to enable the client to explore some flexibility and healthy permeability, such that there would be some chewing and some choiceful ability to take in what was nutritious. It is perhaps worth noticing and noting one complexity here, that to acknowledge a long-standing unmet need is also to come into contact with the profound loss that is often associated with it.

More recently I have a sense that his boundary is becoming less fixed, and food has played a vital role in this, again both metaphorically and literally. Having delivered a cake, one day one of the children of his friends gave his cake tin back with a cup-cake in it. The fact that it was baked by a child mattered. He ate it. This was a defining moment in his ability to begin re- structuring his relationships, his willingness to receive and to acknowledge his needs, the losses and his sense of who he is.

Case study – Ellie

Another example is my client Ellie (pseudonym). She has, in her own words, a difficult relationship with her bodily self. This manifests in various ways, which impact her daily life and her ability to take support from others. This case exemplifies some of the typical boundary disturbances which relate to the process around what is taken in and what can be rejected or metaphorically spat out.

Ellie recalls being a young child who did not like apples. She told her mother, who continued to put them in her lunch box. This was one of many boundary breaches, many of which were in relation to her body. Ellie was expected to swallow what her mother thought was good for her, and she recalls being given no capacity to choose or express any preferences. All meals and food were controlled by her mother. She could never take food from the fridge or help herself to any snacks. All food, portion size and timing of meals was determined by her mother.

Also, no one was allowed in their home. Neither the children nor the parents ever had friends to visit or to stay. She describes numerous of these fixed positions about who or what was allowed in. Similarly, Ellie recalls having no say about who or what was allowed to 'invade' her body. It seems there was no say, no choice, no flexibility. Therefore, she could not develop an ability to really listen to or respond to her bodily sensations, which manifested in significant problems in both being aware of and responding to her needs. She stopped knowing if and when she was hungry or full. This 'desensitization' expanded to include an inability to recognize or respond to pain, both physical and emotional. When she first arrived in therapy, she would often tell me things some time after they occurred and usually when she was already feeling somewhat better. We discussed how this was a pattern in all of her relationships. Although she now has some very good friends, she would typically only share difficulties with them when she was sure that she would not impact them negatively. In other words, she feared breaching their boundaries with something they could not or would not want to hear. She believed that her needs may have a contaminating or poisoning impact on the other. So, although she would receive some support, this invariably came after the original need, and her friends would have no idea about how hard things had been for her. Although she may have shared some detail, she would often make light of it, and then would experience some disappointment that her pain and need went unacknowledged. Over the course of therapy, Ellie is beginning to experiment with how and when she lets me in and keeps me out. She is learning, or re-learning, how to manage her boundaries. We are engaged in a complex dance of offering, chewing, swallowing and spitting. She is discovering how to be aware of her sensations, how to interpret them and what are healthy and choiceful ways to respond them. Like many of us Ellie now eats things she did not like when she was a child, though still no apples.

Case study – Kelly

My final example is a woman Kelly (pseudonym) who came to therapy following witnessing and responding to a traumatic incident. Over the weeks that followed, she was shocked by how much this was impacting her daily life. She could not sleep or eat. As she shared more general information about herself, some interesting patterns began to emerge, including her long-standing erratic eating and her reported complete lack of awareness of hunger and thirst. This was particularly interesting given she had been an international sportswoman, who otherwise was very much in touch with her body, in terms of what 'it' was capable of. In the months that followed, it became clear that she held an unusually high level of responsibility towards others and not towards herself. She came across as highly sensitized towards the needs of others but very desensitized to herself.

Kelly was curious about what we have together named as her somewhat anomalous relationship with her bodily self. As a sportswoman, she would pay close attention to her calorie intake. She reported eating a specific number of calories each day. On reflection she now sees this as somewhat mechanical, rather than responding to sensations. She can, however, recall many positive memories relating to food, including several childhood rituals. She is now interested in how these invariably involve others, and how she can still provide food and engage in food rituals with her family. When she is alone, she reports no sensation of hunger or thirst. The question is, did she dull her sensations as a creative adjustment, so that it became both a habitual and understandable response to her earlier environment? In other words, was it a genuinely creative way to manage her situation? What was she hungry for that was not responded to? Now she often uses language of 'I'm fine', 'it doesn't matter' which is clearly code for 'I don't matter', which can be understood in Gestalt terms as a 'core belief' (Joyce and Sills, 2014). If one does not matter, then there is no point in listening to needs, or anticipating, that needs will be heard by others.

Although over time Kelly has gained significant awareness of how her past is impacting her present, some of these profound responses recur at times. Consequently, we have been exploring this metaphorically, culminating in paying attention to, for example, what of her current situation she feels she cannot swallow.

Chapter summary

The breadth and variety of our human needs bring us into a multitude of interactions with other people, organisms and objects, the natural environment and societal structures. These interactions affect both us as individuals and the other people or environments involved. Life seems to go much better when we can integrate our thoughts, feelings, spiritual expression and our physical bodies. Feeling whole and focused enables us to respond to other people and the wider environment in as resourced a manner as possible. The ease and integrity of this exchange are an indication of mental health.

Activities

Here are some activities for increasing awareness of the contact boundary. The first is for you to explore your individual experience of being an embodied being in a relational world. The second can be tried with one other person, the third with three or more people. Please allow time to reflect on what you experience, and capture it by sharing, writing or drawing.

3.1 Individual

Relax and allow your focus to come to your body. Notice the points of connection with your environment: your weight on a chair, if you are seated; feet maybe touching the ground; the embrace of gravity that allows us to be where we are and still; the feel of your clothes, notice the texture and temperature of the different fabrics that are touching your body; is it different to feel them from the 'inside' from how it feels to touch the 'outside' of them with your hand; the air on your face; maybe a slight tickle from a whisp of hair on your cheek or neck; your nostrils, with seemingly no effort on your part, regulating the exchange of gasses with your environment that keeps you and the world alive; breath following breath; the relative coolness of the air going in contrasting with the relative warmth as it leaves. . . . Where do 'you' end and where does the world begin? Is it different around various parts of your body? Can you find a way to explore how you experience the seam of connection, maybe moving head, hands or feet.

When you are ready, release your attention. Write or draw your responses in a notebook or journal.

3.2 *In twos*

This is an exercise I was given at the beginning of my Gestalt training and I have come across it in various different forms many times over the years. Decide who will go first. This person speaks for 2 minutes, while the other listens in silence (ok to respond with facial expressions). Everything the speaker says has to begin with 'Now I am aware of. . .'. At the end of the time, the listener feeds back whatever they noticed about the awareness of the other. Change over.

3.3 *Group*

Ask everyone in the group to relax and imagine an image coming towards them. Some people may find that a sound or a feeling comes more easily, which is fine. Just take the first thing that comes, however surprising or unlikely. If you have the time and resources, you could ask people to draw or write about what came to them. Otherwise ask everyone to describe what they saw, heard or felt. Afterwards, discuss what this might mean for the group. This is an exercise for the imagination, so it doesn't matter how creative (or outrageous) the ideas become.

Just in case you are wondering why this is relevant, the early stages of the formation of a gestalt involve the imaginative part of our selves. In the process of their emerging, our concerns can arrive in the same manner as they do in dreams, through images and atmospheres. . . . Generally, this is useful because it makes us able to consider a range of possibilities, and we can try some out safely in our imagination, assessing potential outcomes without running the risk of the consequences of acting on them. Your group can explore the process of what is emerging between them at an early stage and increase their understanding of it before taking action, so refining the decision-making process.

I am using this capacity now by imagining you as reader even while I'm in the process of writing the words. . . .

Personal reflection – relationships with food

Liz, who is the illustrator of this book, and I have known each other almost all our lives. Here is something about what the relationship means for me.

In my earliest memories you are there. My mother and me, your mother and you; your mother and my mother, you and me. They had met at primary school, and their birthdays were within four days of each other, in October. This October your mother was 93; my mother died 12 years ago. You and your mother were there at her funeral. But I didn't know you so well then.

You left me twice. First when your family moved out of your grandmother's house, three streets from where my family lived in my grandmother's house. A bus-ride instead of a walk made things more difficult, but we still went to each other's houses all the time. My mother would put me on the bus with the coins for my ticket in my hand and ask the conductor to put me off at the right stop. At the other end, you and your mother would be waiting.

I liked going to your house because your mother made cakes. At mine we had shop bought. I noticed that, somehow despite the cakes, you were very thin. I used to wish I was like you because you could slide the bracelet that was a 'free gift' in the comic we liked over your elbow to your upper arm, which was how it was meant to be worn. With my arm, the bracelet stopped well short of my elbow. You could wear the high-heeled pink plastic toy shoes, that belonged to me, out for a walk, while my feet started to hurt after a few steps.

Our birthdays are within three days of each other, but there is a year between us too. Which meant that, although we went to the same school, we were in different classes, and other friends came into the picture. Then you moved away to a different country. My mother wrote letters to your mother, carefully inscribed to the unfamiliar-sounding address. We had never heard of Worthing.

Then almost a whole lifetime went by. We both married and had a family, although you managed to hold on to your marriage, while I couldn't. By coincidence (or maybe something else) we both trained as psychotherapists. Both of us grandmothers, we meet regularly now. I envy you your front-garden allotment and white AGA. I think you may envy the less intense family demands made on me, because I have fewer children and grandchildren. When we eat in each other's homes, or even when we go out for dinner together, our contrasting relationships with food become apparent. We discuss it a lot together, and accommodate each other's differing needs when we can, understanding that I like potatoes and you definitely don't.

We used to look so different from one another: you dark-haired and skinny, me plump and blonde. Now that I have lost some weight, and we both have greying hair and use glasses sometimes, we seem to have begun to resemble each other. I liked when we were in Abergavenny market and the stall-holder called out 'You look like sisters' and you replied: 'We almost are'.

But not quite. We came back together when your mother was ill. There are not many people left in the world who remember me when I was a child and it seemed terribly important not to let anyone go unremarked. I asked if I could visit her over in Sussex, where you live close by to one another, and you invited me to stay at your house. It was November and the afternoon was already darkening as we walked over to your mother's. She didn't look that different: still very thin, her mannerisms recognizable as those I remember from being a child. Except her hair was white instead of burning auburn. We drank tea, talked a lot about the past and looked at old photographs, and I was pleased I had come. Thankfully she recovered, and we somehow re-membered who we are for one another.

Food note

When a mealtime is approaching, what do you do? The answer probably depends on whether you are the one responsible for providing the food. If that happens to be the case, then how do you respond? I have to say I am the kind of person who likes to plan ahead. I'm usually at home so I shop regularly for basic fresh ingredients that I might need, like fresh vegetables and fruit, milk, eggs, cheese, butter and bread if I haven't baked my own recently. I have frozen fish and peas, and plastic containers with extra portions of meals that I have previously cooked in my freezer. My store cupboard contains tinned tomatoes, some pulses in packets or tins, olive and rapeseed oils, a few different vinegars (like balsamic for salad dressings and wine vinegars for cooking) jars of mayonnaise, pickles and fruit spread. I also have tomato ketchup, which my grandson likes, and which I use if I make my own baked beans (see recipe in the following).

When a mealtime approaches, I'm usually able to find what I want to eat among the provisions I have. Sometimes I follow a recipe. There are so many available on the internet, and I also have shelves of recipe books. While I enjoy some food programmes on television, I find I need a written-down recipe if I'm going to try and cook something I've seen.

An alternative to a recipe is to take what you have available and work out how to make it delicious. This gets easier with practice. Onions and garlic are usually a good base and salt and pepper are the basic condiments for bringing out the flavour of the ingredients you choose. I believe the important thing is to taste. If food tastes good to you, it will probably taste good to others who may be lucky enough to eat it. Trust your own instincts. You will notice how roasting root vegetables in butter tastes differently from roasting them in olive oil. What suits your appetite at this moment?

This is the recipe I use:

www.theguardian.com/lifeandstyle/wordofmouth/2014/may/01/how-to-cook-perfect-baked-beans

References

Berger, J. (1972) *Ways of seeing*. London: BBC and Penguin Books.

Bettelheim, B. (1976) *The uses of enchantment*. London: Penguin Books.

Büber, M. (1958/1984) *I and Thou*. Edinburgh: T. & T. Clark.

Clarkson, P. and Mackewn, J. (1993) *Key figures in counselling and psychotherapy: Fritz Perls* (Series editor Windy Dryden). London: Sage.

Crocker, S.F. (1981) 'Proflection', *Gestalt Journal*, 4(2), pp. 13–34.

Freud, S. (1905) 'On psychotherapy', in Strachey, J. (ed.) *The standard edition of the complete psychological works of Sigmund Freud, Volume 7*. London: Hogarth.

Humphrey, K. (1986) 'Laura Perls: A biographical sketch', *Gestalt Journal*, 9(1), pp. 5–11.

Joyce, P. and Sills, C. (2014) *Skills in gestalt counselling and psychotherapy*. 3rd edn. London: Sage.

Kumar, S. (2017) *Soil, soul, society*. London: Leaping hare Press.

Lewin, K. (1926/1999) 'Intention, will and need', in Gold, M. (ed.) *The complete social scientist: A kurt Lewin reader* (pp. 117–136). Washington, DC: American Psychological Association.

Merleau-Ponty, M. (1964/1968) *The visible and the invisible* (trans. Lingis, A.) Evanston, IL: Northwestern University Press. (Originally published as *Le Visible et L'Invisible*. Paris: Gallimard, 1964).

Perls, F., Hefferline, R.E. and Goodman, P. (1977 [1951]) *Gestalt therapy – Excitement and growth in the human personality*. London: Pelican Books.

Perls, F., Hefferline, R.E. and Goodman, P. (1992) *Gestalt therapy: Excitement and growth in the human personality*. London: Souvenir Press.

Perls, F.S. (1992a) *Ego, Hunger and aggression*. New York: The Gestalt Journal Press.

Perls, L. (1992b) *Living at the boundary*. Gouldsboro, PA: Gestalt Journal Press.

Rovelli, C. (2016) *Seven brief lessons on physics*. UK: Penguin Books.

Sartre, J-P. (1984) *Being and nothingness* (trans. Barnes, H.E.). New York: Washington Square Press.

Stoehr, T. (1994) *Here, now, next*. San Francisco, CA: Gestalt Institute of Cleveland.

Wheeler, G. (1991) *Gestalt reconsidered*. New York: Gardner Press.

Wheeler, G. (1998) *Gestalt reconsidered*. Cambridge, MA: GIC Press.

Wollants, G. (2012) *Gestalt therapy: Therapy of the situation*. London: Sage.

Yontef, G. (1993) *Awareness, dialogue and process: Essays on gestalt therapy*. Highland, NY: Gestalt Journal Press.

5 A world of food

History and current situation

Introduction

Up to now, the main focus of concern has been the individual physiological, emotional and psychological experience of being human in an interconnected world. This exploration has, hopefully, provided an opportunity for readers to develop further insight into the nature and complexity of our human attributes. One aim of this examination has been to identify the essential conditions that contribute to mental health. Feeding our bodies with the appropriate nutrients in a regulated and balanced way is probably one of the main essential conditions, and connects directly with the topic of the book.

As whole beings, we also need to give attention to our thoughts and emotions, and maybe the spiritual aspects of ourselves, if those are significant for us. The ability to direct our thoughts productively, finding ways to avoid dwelling on imaginary catastrophes and developing the resilience to be able to encounter real threats with courage and equanimity, supports us with the inevitable challenges we face. The capacity to feel and express the full range of human emotions also helps us to encounter the difficulties life presents, as well as appreciating the joys. Connection with the transcendent enables us to access and be resourced by a sense of mystery, awe and wonder, whether or not it is associated with organized religion. Identifying and acknowledging the conditions that support us in the full range of our expression as human beings can resource practitioners who work in the field of physical and mental health and wellbeing, whatever their particular context.

As a species, we have evolved in particular ways. In the previous chapters, I have examined some ideas about what it means to be human, emphasizing how interpersonal and situational dynamics influence possibilities and shape the outcomes of interactions. Using the concept of the 'Contact Boundary' (see Chapter 4) as a metaphor for our ongoing experience of being, I have highlighted the close and responsive interface between a person and their world, whether that means other people, non-human beings or the wider environment, including what we eat.

The consuming of a variety of other living constituents that coexist with us in our world – those we call food – brings us nourishment and satisfaction and provides essential nutrients for our bodies and brains. Mealtimes punctuate our days in accordance with the practices our particular cultures have evolved over time

DOI: 10.4324/9781003172161-6

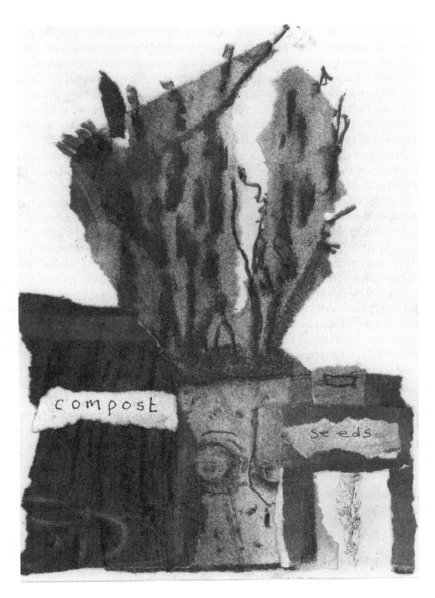

Restoring nourishment

(possibly a very long time), bringing opportunities for rest and pleasure as well as nourishment.

I have described how these foodstuffs are processed by the body in order to produce substances that are necessary for the good functioning of both head and gut brains, and therefore our experience of being alive. Using the important neurotransmitter serotonin as an example, I have identified the food sources of some of the protein, carbohydrate, fats, vitamins and minerals necessary for its production. All being well, these essential substances are found in the constituents of our daily diets. We know that we cannot survive if our brains and bodies are denied this sustenance for any length of time, and yet we are dependent on our environment to make them available. This means that the way our society treats the production and supply of foodstuffs is crucial for all of us.

This chapter changes the direction of the exploration by focusing on the world's relationship with food, which is at least as diverse, complex, multi-faceted and nuanced as those of individuals. Our very lives depend on the system that supplies our food, yet when provisions are abundantly available from early morning to late at night, as they are in supermarkets in the UK and other western countries, it is very easy not to think about that or its implications. Maybe the food industry likes it that way (Steel, 2013). The factors that drive the wider food environment seem, anyway, too remote for us to influence and control. 'Big Ag' (the multi-national companies that control the growing of food) has a force that is exercised across international boundaries, and in the spheres of politics and finance, as well as in direct food production. In this chapter, we will start to explore how some of these dynamics operate and begin to look at other possibilities that may better secure the nutritional quality of our food and possibly point to more wholesome and equitable societal alternatives.

Grounded

Our bodies are complex organisms that need regular access to food to survive and thrive. These foodstuffs are rich and various, delighting us with their textures and flavours, generously inviting us to provide ourselves with the nutrients that sustain us.

The foundation from which these nutrients derive is soil, and it is under threat

An article in the Guardian on 5th December 2020 (p. 9) is headlined:

'Future looks bleak for the soils that underpin life on Earth, warns UN'

The article, written by Damian Carrington, refers to a report from the UN Food and Agriculture Organization that was compiled by 300 scientists. They claim, 'the worsening state of soils is at least as important as the climate crisis'. They describe soil as 'like the skin of the living world, vital but thin and fragile, and easily damaged by intensive farming, forest destruction, pollution and global heating'. They also emphasize that 'few things matter more to humans because we rely on the soil to produce food'. Professor Nico Eisenhauer, who co-authored the report, reminds us that 'soils simultaneously produce food, store carbon and purify water' and observes that many of the microbes involved in transforming waste into nutrients have not yet been studied by scientists and little is known about their contribution to soil quality.

Until I started writing this book, I had not properly understood the connection between the nutrients my brain and body need to continue to function, and the quality of the soil that produces the fruit and vegetables I eat. (The soil that grows the food that the animals providing my milk, cheese and eggs, and that become my meat, have to eat also has an indirect effect on me.) The UN Food and Agriculture Organization has identified that, because of the depletion of the soils on our Earth, there are only 60 harvests left.

See: www.fao.org/soils-2015/events/detail/en/c/338738/.

How will my grandchild's grandchildren, who may be around by then, feed themselves?

The nutrients that keep us alive come from our food. How do they get there? From the soil in which they are grown. In the next section, I describe how modern industrialized farming practices (chemical fertilizer and pesticides) came to be adopted. We know now that these fertilizers prevent the soil from replenishing itself, meaning that more and more chemicals are needed to produce the same amount of crops, so it becomes almost like the cycle of an addiction (Steel, 2013).

Nitrogen, phosphorus and potassium, along with carbon dioxide and water, were considered by early twentieth century agricultural chemists to be the necessary nutrients for plant production. However, they did not take into account the contribution of organic matter both to plant quality and to soil health. In its natural state (or if well kept), organic matter creates a mycorrhizal layer in which fungi and microorganisms create a symbiotic relationship with plant roots. For a more in-depth explanation of this interaction, 'The Hidden Half of Nature' by David R. Montgomery and Anne Biklé is a source that is both accessible and authoritative.

For me, what seems most relevant about the discovery of the significance of the presence of microorganisms in soil is that it parallels the discovery of the significance of microorganisms in our own bodies, and not just in the gut. Although they make up 'half the weight of life on Earth' (Montgomery and Biklé, 2016, p. 25), a lot has yet to be known about the microorganisms that share our world. This is probably because they are too small to see with the naked eye, so the technology of microscopes has needed to reach an appropriate level before they could be studied in detail, and this standard was achieved only towards the end of the twentieth century. This is not to say that their presence was not known about before that. Microorganism (or microbes, both terms seem to mean the same thing) make beer, wine and vinegar, which have all been produced for centuries.

Then what is a microbe? Montgomery and Biklé name five major groups (p. 25):

Archaea.   The oldest form. Resembles a lump of pastry into which someone has pressed the length of their thumb.
Bacteria.   Which look like a very hairy, elongated kiwi fruit with a tail.
Fungi.   Like tiny branches of seaweed.
Protists.   Asymmetric starfish.
Viruses.   Spiny balls, probably more familiar since the Covid-19 pandemic.

These microbes were there at the beginning of life on the earth. Their interactions produced oxygen in the atmosphere and the beginnings of all life, including plants, animals and us. They are found in rocks and water, as well as on skin, lips, eyes and nostrils. Where we live and what we eat change our bodies' microbes. As plant and animal species become extinct, potentially so do the microbes associated with their way of life, and we don't know yet what this might mean for ongoing life (including that of our own species).

Barber (2016, p. 69) mentions species of microbes that are 'so interrelated, so connected to one another and the surrounding ecosystem that studying them individually under a microscope has until very recently been next to impossible'. We cannot remove microorganisms from our bodies to study them because they will not survive apart from us. It seems that these tiny entities are also deeply embedded in their context, just as we humans are. As we understand more about them, maybe we as a species will come to appreciate our interconnectedness at a more visceral level. We are never quite alone because we have our microbiome with us!

This invisible, interconnected world of microorganisms is essential for both producing and digesting the food we eat. Returning to the discussion of the role of plants in this ecosystem brings us back to the crucial importance of soil, and its fragility. The word 'soil' is not the same as the word 'land', although they are connected. Soil can be touched and felt with the hand, it has an individual smell. it is human somehow in scale. By contrast, land is impersonal, untenable . . . Maybe I think this way because my personal connection with land has generally meant having a garden, and access to public open spaces and countryside. I have worked with farmers and, without generalizing too much, I comprehend that their relationship is different. Their land somehow gives them freedom, although their time is commandeered by the need to do the work that maintains the system it supports. Land and a sense of self can become inextricably intertwined in those circumstances.

Land is also a commodity. Kumar (2017, p. 138) observes,

> Land, Labour and Capital, the principles of classical economics, have been turned upside down by modern economics. . . . In this model, land and labour exist to serve capital. . . . In modern economics, money has become the wealth – whereas money should be considered merely a measure of wealth, a means of exchange and not wealth itself.

It seems that, in order to resolve the problems connected with the nourishment of our minds and bodies, we may need to re-consider capitalism as an economic system. In present times, capitalism goes hand-in-hand with neoliberalism, which has been the dominant political framework in the west since the late twentieth century. The spheres of food production and distribution are inextricably involved with economics and politics. I return to the consequences of this later in the chapter, but first some historical background.

A brief history of the world in foodstuffs

How did we arrive at a situation where we are destroying the environment that nourishes us? And how can we have adopted a system by means of which many people in our world are hungry, while others are overfed? Here is a short summary of the development of our relationship with food as a species. For a deeper and more detailed discussion, Carolyn Steel's (2020) book 'Sitopia' is an invaluable resource.

Hunter-gatherers

In 'Catching Fire' (2010), Biological Anthropologist Richard Wrangham argues that the development of humans into the species we recognize ourselves to be today is connected with the ability to cook our food. Raw food is much more difficult to eat and digest, so eating cooked food has meant that our bodies have developed differently from those of other primates, like the chimpanzees and gorillas who still eat their food raw. Our mouths, teeth and jaws have become comparatively smaller, and so has our digestive system. Wrangham believes that the ability to manage with smaller digestive systems made energy available for the development of larger brains.

Groups of hunter-gatherers would be composed of 30 to 60 people (Steel, 2020). Each member would know the other people in the group personally and have an ongoing relationship over time. Wrangham observes that the greater intelligence consequent from the development of larger brains would have been helpful for negotiating the web of relationships in these more complex social groups. The development of co-operation among people has been intrinsic to the evolution of society towards what we recognize as our experience today. As tribes gathered around the campfire to share the spoils of the day's hunt, or distribute the roots, leaves and berries that had been harvested from their surrounding landscape, they are likely to have practised similar behaviours and attitudes to those we use around our own tables in the twenty-first century. To live in community, whether it is a family, a neighbourhood or a nation, it is necessary to trust that (in the main) all members will follow commonly agreed norms. The norms around eating are fundamental because mealtimes are participated in at regular intervals, holding significant aspects of the culture of the group, as well as keeping all members as alive and healthy as is possible in the circumstances. We begin to learn these norms as soon as we can sit up and join in a meal.

For their own survival and wellbeing, early humans would have needed to evolve ways of maintaining cohesion by sanctioning behaviours that undermined the good functioning of society. What 'good-functioning' looked like was likely to have been decided by a privileged group (Wrangham, 2010). Some of the ways that developed then to cope with dynamics of status and power still exist in the twenty-first century: the equivalent of going out to hunt still has higher status than staying at home to forage and nurture. The gender inequalities implicit in this system will be explored in the next chapter.

Farming

Around 12,000 years ago, in the 'Fertile Crescent' of the Middle East, people began to gather seeds from wild grasses and process it to make flour. In order to harvest the grain at the right time, the former wanderers had to settle (Steel, 2013). Rather than collecting what was available and eating it on the same day, it became possible to store food and consume it sometime later. 'It is hard to overstate the impact of farming on human history' (Steel, 2020, p. 93). Agriculture offered stability so that, 'poetry, pottery and counting ensued, followed by architecture, institutions and eventually cities' (p. 94). The security that the ability to store food provided gave opportunities for the making of objects that then did not have to be carried from place to place, and possibilities for other creative pursuits. The complexity of managing the production and distribution processes of the stored foodstuffs required the development of writing and counting. Money started to come into use when it became convenient to have a way of transferring ownership of goods other than by direct barter. The first traces of this currency were found in Sumer in the third millennium BCE (Steel, 2020, p. 239). Banking began in Amsterdam in 1609 (Steel, 2013, p. 141).

When there are goods, the idea of possession becomes relevant. When considerable time and effort needs to be invested in maintaining the soil, producing the plants and processing and storing the harvest, the matter of the ownership of land begins to become significant too. The question of who owned the land, and who worked on it, along with the production of enough food to feed the population, continued to shape how societies organized themselves. In Britain, by the end of the seventeenth century, philosopher John Locke was giving some thought to the ethics of how this process was evolving in response to questions about the nature of land ownership at that time. Steel sums his ideas up in this way: 'It followed that if a farmer tilled the land, he earned the right to call it his own. However (and here was the rub), this was only true *provided each man took only what he needed*, (italics in original) and no more' (2013, p. 27). The right to share in the world's resources came with the responsibility to take only as much as was needed, according to Locke, but that idea never really caught on at the time, and doesn't seem to have yet.

The need to feed a growing population led to an agrarian revolution in Britain in the eighteenth century. The 'feudal system', with a lord of the manor, and serfs to work on the land had become outdated. The large open fields, with separate strips of land that had been cultivated for the benefit of the peasants themselves, as well as their lords, disappeared. The land was enclosed into the smaller, hedge-bound landscapes that are still familiar to us now. Deprived of the means of making their bread, many country-dwellers moved into the growing towns.

The need to produce food shapes the landscape of the countryside and the lives of the population. New farming methods, which seemed to be able to increase production, were introduced when they became available. Steel (2013, p. 38) tells the story of Justus von Liebig, a German chemist who created the first fertilizer in 1836. Having initially achieved success, as time went on it became clear that the natural fertility of the land was disturbed by chemical fertilizers, and more and more additives were necessary to maintain yields. 'I have sinned against the Creator' was Liebig's conclusion at the end of his life.

Steel goes on to describe the consequences of commercial farming techniques in the USA at the beginning of the twentieth century. The ethos of the founding fathers of the new country was the belief that investing time and effort into the land was essential for the right to possess it. The native inhabitants' very different values system, of serving the land rather than exploiting it, meant that their ancestral grounds were taken from them as the new country evolved. Settlers, mainly from Europe, moved in and set about producing as much grain as possible. Initially, high yields plus the introduction of the railroads and innovative packing techniques created very lucrative business opportunities. Subsequently, the combination of intensive farming methods and drought led to a situation known as the 'Dust Bowl' during which, being by now without its organic infrastructure, the topsoil just blew away, leaving the settlers with no choice but to move on and find work elsewhere (Steel, 2013, p. 39).

In post-war Britain, the need to feed the population led to the 1947 Agriculture Act, which permitted the use of the pesticide DDT (dichlorodiphenyltrichloroethane), which decimated insect life, depleting the birds, which fed on insects, and also threatening the human food chain. After a public outcry following the publication in 1962 of 'Silent Spring' by Rachel Carson, DDT was banned in the USA and Europe. It is still being used in parts of the developing world with predictably devastating results (Steel, 2013, p. 41).

Other food calamities in the UK related to modern farming practices include traces of the harmful salmonella bacterium being found in eggs in 1988, BSE or 'mad-cow' disease in 1992 and the foot and mouth epidemic in 2001. Steel concludes an analysis of the current situation in this devastating way.

> During the second half of the twentieth century, global food production increased by 145 per cent – the equivalent of 25 per cent extra per person worldwide – yet 850 million people face hunger every day. It doesn't make much sense, but then very little about the food industry does.
>
> (Steel, 2013, pp. 43–44)

Cities

When people came to live in cities, the connection with the land that produced the food needed to sustain the population was broken. Historically, cities have dealt with the problem of feeding urban populations in different ways: ancient

Rome brought in supplies from its empire by ship. The navigability of the Thames meant that London has always been able to bring food into the heart of the city. Pre-industrial Paris, on the other hand, had to find alternative ways of transporting food, bringing it in from the countryside on barges and carts (Steel, 2020). Even when a city was able to feed itself adequately from its agricultural hinterland, there was still a desire for imported goods. These might include items that could not be produced locally because of climate or season. In the UK, this might involve olive oil and wine, and other speciality or luxury products. Imported items could also be those that cost less to buy from other countries than to grow at home, like the American grain produced in the early twentieth century in the boom that preceded the Dust Bowl. The UK still imports fruit and vegetables that could be grown locally and that are in season here, although this may not continue very much longer, either for political reasons or because environmental constraints, like a shortage of water, may affect producers (Steel, 2013).

Geography and accessibility initially limited the growth of cities. Keeping foodstuffs fresh and edible as they made the journey from the countryside where they were produced to the city where they were consumed was an issue. Different commodities had their particular challenges. Grain was transported by horse-drawn carts and in barges, but it was vulnerable to rotting and pests on the journey. Animals such as cattle and geese walked from their farms to the cities where they would eventually be eaten, driven along special highways, separate from those used by regular traffic (Steel, 2013). The echoes of these 'Drovers' Ways' are still observable in the Welsh landscape in the names of roads and the names of pubs.

The transport of milk from cow to consumer had been such an unwholesome process that many people avoided using milk altogether. From the mid-nineteenth century, with the arrival of the railways, transport between countryside and city became quicker and easier, allowing cities to spread. The idea of the 'milk-train' came into being, bringing an air of the countryside into the city along with the day's fresh milk (Steel, 2013). I still remember the first train of the day between London and Cardiff being called the milk-train, although it probably isn't any more. . .

With the arrival of supermarkets in the mid-twentieth century, the provision of necessary items became big business. Now, in the third decade of the twenty-first century, the systems that provide the staple food supply of most of us in the west, and certainly here in the UK, are in the hands of global conglomerates that control the whole of the food supply chain. They are powerful enough to influence government and to ignore any laws that don't suit them by being well able to afford any fines they might accrue. They are sufficiently powerful that they can pay farmers pretty much what they like and force them to accept processes and procedures that suit their own requirements (Steel, 2013).

Instead of carts and sailing vessels, container ships and lorries transport the goods. Steel (2013, p. 65) describes one of the country's main transport hubs at Crick, close to the small town of the same name in the English Midlands. She draws a vivid picture of the size of the enterprise, and the constant activity of the lorries to-ing and fro-ing around it, the whole operation governed by sophisticated computer systems that respond to the purchase of every single, individual item taken from the supermarket shelf. This replenishment system is called 'just-in-time' and avoids the need for storage, which is costly. It also contributes to addressing the need for keeping food fresh and edible on the journey from producer to consumer, often over very long distances. This precision-driven operation is supported by sophisticated systems of logistics and involves the use of packaging techniques that enhance product freshness. The distance vehicles covered in support of this effort in one year – 2002 – amounts to the same as travelling all the way around the world 750,000 times. The only thing about this system of distribution for our foods is that, as Steel, observes, 'Most of it doesn't taste as nice as it might have done straight out of the ground, but since most of us rarely eat fresh food, we've forgotten what it's supposed to taste like anyway' (2013, p. 63).

Money and value, labour and land

Unless you produce most of your own food, then you will probably use money to meet the cost of your mealtimes. The amount of money you have available to you has significance for what, how much and, maybe, how you eat. When I was a child, most of the available money went on feeding the family. I was nearly 5 before my parents and I moved out of my grandmother's place and into a home of our own, because my parents had to save for years in order to be able to afford it. Nowadays, I'm still used to prioritizing food on the table and a roof over my head, even though the society around me is so much more affluent. These days, I can afford to buy staple foodstuffs as well as regular 'treats', like artisan cheese, organic free-range eggs and high-quality chocolate biscuits, as well as seasonal organic vegetables. At the same time, I am seeing and hearing about families whose level of income is such that they have to find the cheapest possible foods to feed themselves and their children, often not having enough and so going without. Others are needing free school meals in order to survive, and food banks have plenty of take up. How can it be that there is so much inequality in one of the richest countries in the world?

Certainly, one reason is the economic system used in the UK, as well as in large parts of the developed world. Capitalism involves individual ownership of resources by certain people, and the participation of others in those enterprises by providing labour in return for some kind of monetary reward. The Agricultural Revolution that began in the UK in the eighteenth century meant that the ordinary people moved out of the countryside and into cities. There, they began working in factories, and other places, in return for a financial wage, which could then be used to buy food and lodgings for the worker's use. Rather than their producing food for themselves directly, a financial transaction was involved.

The land that they had left was enclosed into smaller, hedge-bound fields that became privately owned by an elite class. The earlier system had involved stretches of common land being available to the whole community, where everyone had a right to use the resources they found there to provide food and shelter for themselves. Enclosure changed that significantly, although not quite everything fell into private ownership at that time. There are still some stretches of common land in existence in Britain now, varying a lot in their particular natures.

Two examples of them are especially familiar to me. The closer one to where I live now is Llantrisant Common, a large area of grassland in mid-Glamorgan, where sheep still graze, and mushrooms can be harvested in the autumn. Apart from the locals who graze and gather, people drive there to walk their dogs, take bike rides or just enjoy the open space, being surrounded otherwise by buildings and roads in an area that is highly populated.

The second example is Ealing Common in West London. The busy North-Circular Road borders one edge, and the 207 bus service travels (along with cars, lorries, many other buses and, actually, some bikes) up and down the almost equally busy Uxbridge Road that intersects it. This thoroughfare passes right through the middle of the common land, which means that walkers have to cross a main road to go from one side to the other. Despite the heavy traffic and general busy-ness, it is still a pleasant green interlude among all the shops and houses. More than that, I have seen people perform 'Tree-dressing' ceremonies there. These involve tying ribbons around growing trees and speaking words of acknowledgement, praise and promise to them. They are a kind of pagan precursor of Christmas, taking place at winter solstice. I remember seeing circuses there in the summer, too, and parked cars with courting couples after dark.

However common or publicly owned land is used, it provides something significant for its visitors and inhabitants, whether they are human or other-than-human. To call it an amenity reduces it to something mundane and transactional, whereas, actually, it is nourishing, uplifting and maybe even sanctifying. These public spaces, valuable though they are, do not represent a large proportion of the land in Britain. Much of that remains in private ownership and so reflects aspects of the capitalist system. Steel observes: 'One third of all land in Britain, for example, is owned by the aristocracy, one of the factors that perpetuates the structural inequalities of our society' (2020, p. 220).

Back in the eighteenth century, factories, and other money-making ventures that provided work for the population that was leaving the land, were being set up by investors. These were people who had sufficient spare money, after they had met their subsistence requirements, to be able to participate in business activities. While the people with plentiful resources provided the capital, those who needed to earn a wage to feed and sustain themselves provided the labour. The capitalist system developed over time, but one fundamental facet of it has always been the relationship between capital and labour. The Trade Unions evolved as a way of balancing up the power differentials, using the collective power of the workers to negotiate with the financially powerful owners. By the mid to late twentieth century, the Trade Unions had become strong, and not only in privately owned companies. They were also very powerful in the so-called 'nationalized industries' like gas and electric power, the railways and coal production. These organizations, having been considered essential to the general good, had previously been taken into public ownership in the interest of the security of the population. That was about to change.

I remember the year of the miners' strike in 1984/1985. Living in South Wales, I was close to it, although not directly affected. I worked at British Gas at the time and one of my close colleagues was living with a striking miner, so I heard about the difficulties they were having to cope with for many months at first hand. The strike ended a year after it had begun, and without achieving its aims. I watched on television as the miners marched back to work behind their banners, with their heads held proudly high. But their cause had been defeated and the coal industry slowly declined. Mrs Thatcher went on to de-nationalize all the previously nationalized industries, including British Gas. As an employee at the time, I benefitted from an allocation of shares in the newly privatized company, plus the possibility of buying more shares at a concessionary rate, which I did. The intention of the politicians at the time was that ordinary working people (like me) could become shareholders, participating in the capital strand of the system and receiving returns on our investments, in addition to being paid for providing our labour. For some people, those with sufficient spare resources at the right time, this may have been an effective strategy. But those that could not participate were even further left out. Saint Matthew's Gospel in the Christian Bible says, 'For to everyone who has will more be given, and he will have abundance; but from him who has not, even what he has will be taken away' V. 25–29.

With the decline of power in the Trade Unions, and the establishment of capitalism as the dominant economic system, the balance of power shifted between those who provided the labour and those who provided the money. Eventually, this led to what is now known as 'the gig economy', with its resultant lack of security and stability for the workers involved. The political system that accompanied the development of capitalism is neoliberalism. Both these approaches assume that 'the market' is a natural regulator of supply and demand, cost and value. Competition is inherent to the system, and the focus is on the individual entrepreneur rather than on society as a whole. The workings of the market seem inherently designed to result in a dynamic of 'boom and bust'. One relatively recent consequence of the way it operates was the financial crisis in 2008, a contributing factor of which was the way dealers in sub-prime mortgages used financial packages called derivatives.

Nowadays, one quarter of the world's food is traded digitally. The trade is structured as derivatives called 'futures'. These were meant to protect the farmer from price fluctuations caused by lack or glut in the harvest, but the outcome of their adoption is that, 'instead of buying a commodity for its use, one could simply gamble on its future price' (Steel, 2020, p. 124). No wonder the trading arms of big banks have become known as 'casino-banks'. Worryingly, this is reminiscent of the kind of trading that contributed to the crash of 2008. The consequence of that was a period of what was called 'austerity' in the UK, introduced as the political response to the crisis. The detrimental effects of that strategy for the provision of services to the people in society who needed them, including those related to the NHS, were still being felt before the arrival of the pandemic. If a similar crash happened in food trading, then the consequences are almost unthinkable. It has been my own experience over the last few years that the unthinkable can easily happen. First there was Brexit, then the election of Donald Trump in the USA instead of Hillary Clinton. I know I would have been influenced by my own political preferences, but these two occurrences came as an unpleasant shock to me. Then there was the Covid-19 pandemic, which came as a shock to everybody.

Over time, the whole system, both financial and political, has led to inequality. We are now in the position where 1% of the population possesses most of the money and power. There is something very out-of-balance about this system of distribution, and very far from Locke's ideal of taking only as much as is needed. **Many economists now recognize how broken the system is** (Mason, 2015; Raworth, 2017).

In Chapter 7, we will look at some possible approaches to change. Before that, there is one more aspect of our society's relationship with food that needs to be discussed.

Waste

If we were able to avoid waste, there would be enough for everyone, without destroying the natural resources of the planet in order to produce still more. Seventeenth-century philosopher John Locke thought this way about people who waste food: 'if fruits rotted or the venison putrified before he could spend it, he offended against the common law of nature, and was likely to be punished' (Locke, 1690 in Stuart, 2009, p. 5). Our punishment as a society for breaking the common law of nature is grave indeed because the results of our choices are that our continuing existence as a species is becoming more and more questionable.

In our society, many things are wasted. Rare metals are used in electronic devices that start to work less efficiently after a few years and so need to be replaced, often coinciding with a new generation of whatever device it is becoming available. It is often more economical to throw away broken household appliances and buy new ones, than it is to repair them. When I called in a repair company to look at my broken washing machine last year, it cost almost a quarter of the price of a replacement appliance, and they couldn't fix it anyway, so I had to pay for both the repair-person's time and a new machine. I probably have enough clothes to last for the remainder of my lifetime, but I'm still tempted to buy something new when I see an interesting style that I think would suit me. . .

Food waste is an area for particular concern because food is essential for life in a way that mobile phones, washing machines and new jumpers are not. Situations connected with food are where inequalities can become staggeringly obvious, like when homeless people sit at the doors of supermarkets, and also hidden because much of the hunger in the world takes place in countries many of us in the west are unlikely to visit.

The statistics around food waste read like screaming headlines. This link leads to where the UN identifies that **one-third of the food that is produced in the world is wasted.**

www.fao.org/food-loss-and-food-waste/flw-data)#:~:text=One%2Dthird%20of%20food%20produced,1.3%20billion%20tonnes%20per%20year.

For many of us, food seems cheap and plentiful, so it can be easy not to value it very much. Yet the true cost is way more than the price we pay. Food is expensive to produce in terms of natural resources like land and water, and the disposal of food waste is costly both financially and environmentally.

- The food industry is responsible for 30% of greenhouse gas emissions: https://feedbackglobal.org/knowledge-hub/food-waste-scandal/.

- The production of food requires water. This website claims that 25% of the available water in the world is used to produce food that is wasted. https://journals.plos.org/plosone/article?id=10.1371/journal.pone.0007940.

In his book 'Waste' (2009), Tristram Stuart identifies how and where waste occurs:

- On the farm, growers are required to reject vegetables that do not meet the required size and shape specifications.
- In shops, from the disposal of food that has passed its sell-by date.
- In the fishing industry, meeting size and quota requirements for the catch.

These issues have become familiar since Stuart's book was published. Retailers have made an effort to sell 'wonky vegetables', and food that has passed its sell-by-date is given to charities for distribution to the people who need it. Despite these efforts, the system that requires uniformity and constant availability is still in place. Perhaps now that the UK has left the EU, regulations that result in waste can be reviewed, although I'm not hopeful that will happen without a fundamental change of attitude amongst all of us, government and people.

There may be little that we as individuals can do in the face of powerful vested interest, but there is one context in which we have full agency – our own homes. Over half of food waste takes place in the home. See: www.lovefoodhatewaste.com/why-save-food.

What would it take to substantially reduce household food waste? As far as I'm concerned, recognizing it as a significant issue and making the avoidance of waste a priority might be a good starting place. Our busy lives may make that seem challenging, but we don't have to do everything at once. Here are some lessons I have learned over the years:

- Small, incremental changes are more sustainable.
- Beware of offers that encourage me to buy more than I need (however tempting the bargain!).
- Use the available refuse facilities appropriately. In my area, we have food waste bags that go to a central depot to be made into compost, mixed recycling of paper, glass, cans, etc., and black bag waste that goes to landfill. I try to use the appropriate places for items, even if it takes some effort, separating cellophane and cardboard, for example.
- Meet the standards required for recycled waste, like washing out yoghurt pots.
- Work out an attitude to 'sell-by' dates that is comfortable for you, and appropriate for your family. I am very willing to trust how an item smells and looks, maybe even tasting a tiny morsel, and quite happy to eat what still seems wholesome after it has passed its 'sell-by' date. I am more wary about this if I am feeding my grandson than I would be if it was only myself or other adults involved. I have not had any problems with my approach, so I feel confident. If you feel less confident, pay attention to that. I have no scientific proof of this, but I think our bodies have a deep wisdom about what seems appetizing for us and is therefore good to eat.

- Learn how to revive (or camouflage) veg that has begun to look a bit tired. Soaking leafy greens (or root veg that has gone a bit soft) in a big basin of cold water can really make a difference. Otherwise, chopping whatever it is up and putting it into soup is another way for me of making the best of the nutritional value I have paid for.
- Learn how to use leftovers. This is about how to store them safely and also about how to cook or otherwise use them. I put my leftovers into plastic boxes, leaving the lid off until the item is completely cold, so that steam does not condense inside. When it is cold, I put the lid on the box tightly and place it in the fridge, if I know I am going to use it over the next few days. If I want to keep it for longer, I put a sticky label describing the contents on the lid and put it in the freezer. More about cooking leftovers in the 'Food Note' at the end of the chapter.
- Make friends with breadcrumbs. I put any leftover bread into the food-processor, and then keep the crumbs in plastic bags in the freezer. I have a few favourite recipes that use them, often involving frying the breadcrumbs, with the addition of crushed garlic, or a spice, in olive oil until golden and then scooping the mixture onto roasted vegetables. If you don't feel confident to experiment just yet, an internet search for a recipe will probably result in something you might like.

There would be no need to tear up the rainforest to produce palm oil or tear out the mineral infrastructure of the ancestral lands in Australia if all of us were more thoughtful about waste.

Surviving a pandemic – a societal case study

Producing a book that I hope will be useful to readers for many years to come involves making choices about how to treat topics that are current at the time of writing. I want to avoid the danger of focusing on events that may seem currently significant but quickly become stale. I am certain that the 2020 Covid pandemic will shape our attitudes well into the future, so it does seem valid to mention it specifically, particularly because so much of what has happened while we have been facing it has been connected with food. As this chapter is about societal relationships with food, it seems appropriate to give some attention to our shared experience, as events have been unfolding that seemed inconceivable only a year ago. I am writing this in early March 2021 and the vaccine is in full roll-out in the UK, giving us the opportunity to have a 'roadmap' for finally coming out of lockdown.

I want to go back to the beginning, 16th March 2020, almost a year ago. We all stayed at home. Except, of course, people working in the NHS, who became the lauded 'front-line' against the threat of plague, starvation and societal breakdown. Actually, societal breakdown has been more than just a threat. Health and education closed down for the most part, except to keep essential Covid-related services going. Some people were 'furloughed', paid for not working. Others moved their work on-line. I was one of those. I had been meeting clients face-to-face at my home, but the sessions suddenly transferred on to Skype, FaceTime and Zoom. I was surprised at how smooth and easy the transition was.

The announcement to close inessential retail meant that only food shops remained open. Distancing rules made it necessary to queue outside supermarkets, although mandatory mask-wearing had not become part of our daily lives. Some small shops set up barriers between the people serving and customers, and one-way systems to separate shoppers from one another. Others shut up shop entirely and did on-line ordering and deliveries. Pasta, tinned tomatoes and toilet rolls became scarce. Flour disappeared completely from shelves as people took up baking.

Part of the population had unprecedented time and leisure, others faced death, sickness and trauma, and the necessity for and scarcity of PPE (Personal Protective Equipment). Still others, those working in food retail and other essential services, risked exposure to the virus (and the consequences of other people's fear and frustration) for the whole of their work day. Some people were working at their regular job on-line and simultaneously home schooling their children, which was an impossible sleight of hand to which governments seemed oblivious.

We began by thinking of Covid-19 as a great leveller, but we quickly recognized that people who were already disadvantaged by living in inadequate housing in overcrowded neighbourhoods and working in insecure jobs were more likely to catch the disease and also to be negatively affected by the restrictions imposed because of it. It soon became apparent that people of colour were being affected disproportionately. Then there was the situation with free school meals for children from poorer backgrounds. After the intervention of a young professional footballer called Marcus Rashford, the eventual decision was taken to provide them over the summer holiday, as well as in term time. Subsequently, there has been a controversy around the quality and quantity of the food being provided.

The kinds of issues I have been noticing with my clients over the year have reflected the general situation. Some people have faced challenges directly around eating as all the disruption and uncertainties have unfolded. Others have experienced a hiatus: the impossibility of carrying on with their lives as they had planned. Meaninglessness, isolation and boredom have been challenging for many. Others have been exposed to the possibility of infection and having to cope with changes to working practices. At the beginning of the first lockdown, a few of the people I meet who were involved with the NHS described how difficult it had been for them to buy food. By the end of their work day, supermarket shelves had been emptied. I understood well the need for special food provision for these essential workers and was happy to see that local restaurant owners quickly stepped in to provide it.

As thing begin to open up again, we will all have to start to rebuild the shattered economy, decide our priorities as a society and work out a strategy for going forward for ourselves, our families and communities. The inequalities in our society have been made starkly plain as a consequence of the pandemic. People who are overweight, those with diabetes and other chronic physical conditions, and older members of the population have all been experiencing higher levels of risk from the possibility of becoming ill with the virus. Good general health has felt like a source of security. The employment sectors most badly hit, hospitality in particular, involve younger workers: there are children, like my grandson, who don't know what it's like to go to a café because they haven't been available for the majority of their lives. How can we create secure, meaningful work for all our young people going forward?

We all have our 'Covid Stories'. This has been an extract from mine. It has touched on the crucial importance of the food supply chain. Any threats to that and fear, leading to irrational, self-serving behaviour, happens almost at once. Poverty and hunger are linked in this country in a way that I personally find shameful. The link between good nutrition (avoiding obesity and physical conditions that are known to be linked to diet, and particularly to processed food) and resilience to disease has been thrown into high relief. Food is fundamental to the way we operate as a society, as well as affecting our individual mental and physical health.

Now, we probably all need a holiday. We are not sure when that will be possible, but we know we are on the brink of change. What happens now really matters.

Chapter summary

The history of our relationship with food as a species is full of milestones that mark the path to where we are now. From earliest times, the people who have the power to make the rules influence what is available and to whom. The system has identified those who grow and cook and serve, and those who have ownership and are served, and differentiated us from one another. This deep inequality has led us to the stage we are at now, where some of the inhabitants of our world are hungry, while others of us waste all the surplus that we have available to us. With my own personal history, it is difficult for me to acknowledge this, but eating more food than an individual needs is also waste.

The food producers continue to grow more and more food that no one will eat, and the capitalist economic system goes on aiming to create more and more money, for the benefit of those who already have more than they could possibly need. The effect of this exploitation on our planet, on the earth that sustains us and the air that makes us one breathing community means that ours is one of the many species that may become extinct before many more generations have passed.

For practitioners who work facilitatively with others, this sombre situation demands our attention with various degrees of force. We may work with people who struggle to afford food for themselves and their children, while we are comfortably off by comparison. What does it mean for the dynamic in the room in these circumstances? How is it when some really worthwhile change is possible on account of our work, but the resources that would make it a reality are not available? This problem of inequality and exploitation of resources belongs to us all, however much or little we may benefit from it. This reality, and the urgency of finding a different way forward, is very likely to trouble our mental health, and that is probably absolutely appropriate. Although the situation is dire, there are people who are thinking about the way forward and beginning to put changes in place. The next two chapters takes a look at some of those innovators.

Activities

Please consider the following questions. This may involve thinking about them, meditating on them or making a piece of free-flowing, uncensored writing, similar to those in a personal journal.

5.1 Individual

If you were involved with finding a solution to all these societal issues, what kind of future would you envisage for the world?

Journal for 5 minutes, or however long you think you need.

5.2 Two people

If there was some kind of crash on world food markets, what would you miss most?

5.3 Group

I'm inviting you to replicate something of the workshop experience I describe in the 'Personal Reflection' in the following. Discuss with a small group of people, family, colleagues or clients where appropriate:

'How can we talk about the growing and distribution of food in our society without despair or denial, guilt, shame or blame?'

Personal reflection – despair and denial

Years ago, before climate change became undeniable, I remember signing up for a drama workshop held by some people in my then local community who were concerned about its impact. In those days, we used to talk about despair and denial as being typical reactions to the enormity of the climate challenge. The purpose of this workshop was to explore how it might be possible to talk about these issues without evoking either of those responses.

I remember one of the activities we tried that day very vividly. The task was to improvise being a group of people who were talking about food three decades in the future. In the scenario we were asked to envisage, most of what was left by that time was plastic. Our group began imagining how it would be to have to eat plastic and our expressions became those of disgust and longing. 'Remember fish?' I found myself saying, vividly recalling the taste and texture of a mouthful of cod. The half-dozen faces of the other group members all turned towards me and we were silent for a moment. We knew then that the sea was fragile. Now we know the land is fragile too. Also, nearly two of the three future decades we were imagining back then have already slipped by.

In addition to despair and denial, other feelings, like guilt, shame and blame, are probably inevitable sometimes. Yet, in order to move on, we need to be able at least to start acknowledging the emotional fallout of our situation and sharing that understanding with one another. At that workshop, which seems quite a long time ago now, we identified that telling stories might be a gentler and more palatable way of communicating climate-related concerns. I suppose David Attenborough arrived at that understanding too. Maybe, as Socrates implied, it is more enabling to feel part of the solution, rather than part of the problem.

Food note

There are many different kinds of leftovers. I like to cook a big batch of a recipe, eat one portion on the day and put the other, usually three or five portions, in plastic storage boxes to cool and maybe to freeze, depending on the supplies of other things I have at the time. The word 'plastic' has just jumped out at me, probably after having just written the previous section. I feel like I have to say in my own justification that my stock of plastic boxes has been recycled many times. Some of them are more than 20 years old, but still do the job. I also wash out and re-use plastic food bags and sheets of aluminium foil. I have a drawer in my kitchen where the bags and foil sit neatly folded until I need them. Also in the drawer are the brown paper bags that survived their first use clean and whole enough to be used again, and rubber bands, wound around each other into something by now the size of a tennis ball. Probably more than I will ever need in my life, but you never can tell.

Alongside freshly cooked food specifically intended for another time, there are other kinds of leftovers. In my mind, the way leftover food is categorized changes according to whether it has been on somebody's individual plate or not. I am a lot more circumspect if it has been on a plate, so I serve up what I think is enough for the current meal and keep the rest of what I have cooked to the side in case anyone wants more. If not, then it is the usual plastic box and fridge procedure. I think carefully about anything left on someone's plate when we have all finished eating. If it is seemingly untouched and suitably succulent, I will probably keep it; otherwise, it is useful to have my daughter's dog around, who enjoys a modest amount of human food with her own dry feed.

References

Barber, D. (2016) *The third plate*. London: Abacus.
Kumar, S. (2017) *Soil, soul, society*. London: Leaping hare Press.
Locke, J. (1690) 'Second treatise of government', in *Two treatises of government*. London: A. Churchill.
Mason, P. (2015) *Postcapitalism*. UK: Penguin Random House.
Montgomery, D.R. and Biklé, A. (2016) *The hidden half of nature*. London: Norton & Co.
Raworth, K. (2017) *Doughnut economics*. London: Random House Business.
Steel, C. (2013) *Hungry city*. London: Vintage Books.
Steel, C. (2020) *Sitopia*. London: Chatto & Windus.
Stuart, T. (2009) *Waste*. UK: Penguin Random House.
Wrangham, R. (2010) *Catching fire*. London: Profile Books.

6   Difference and diversity

Introduction

Faced with the realities of climate change, the declining nutritional quality of the soil and fundamental, seemingly structural, inequalities among people, how can we go forward? The Covid-19 pandemic is fresh in our minds, and we are still dealing with the emotional and financial fallout from it. As individuals, we may feel confused, vulnerable and powerless in the face of unexpected events and dominant global vested interests. We as practitioners, our families, and our clients too are all being affected by the food that is available to us. Our bodies and brains are coping with the individual nutritional deficits (and excesses) we experience in ways that are more or less successful, depending on individual and environmental factors. This is likely to affect our mental health whether we are aware of it or not.

I believe there is some caution needed when considering mental health issues at a time of world crisis. Many years ago, near the start of my training, people were worried that psychotherapy might address the inner resilience of an individual so successfully that it diminished their impetus to take action to change detrimental situations in the world. Neutralizing people's natural responses to the conditions in which they find themselves is probably not helpful, and possibly unethical, to my mind. Encouraging conformity with societal norms has also been a concern in the context of the purpose and practice of psychotherapy. Thank heavens people are no longer 'treated' in an effort to 'cure' their sexuality. As psychotherapists, we know that we can consider our own cultural norms as 'normal' and then try to impose them on people who have different cultural norms (Littlewood and Lipsedge, 1989). A very wise colleague of mine, who comes from a different cultural background, once said to me as I was well-meaningly trying to explain to her about how Indian cooking had become integrated in British cuisine, 'Let me have my difference' (Kaur, 2010).

Much of what follows is about possible changes for society that may help make a difference to our individual (and collective) sense of wellbeing. Personal change is hard, societal change is even more complex and difficult. In this chapter, we will examine some approaches that may help with understanding the dynamics of large-scale change. Hopefully, this kind of broader knowledge can increase the variety of options available to us as individuals and to the smaller groups in which we participate.

DOI: 10.4324/9781003172161-7

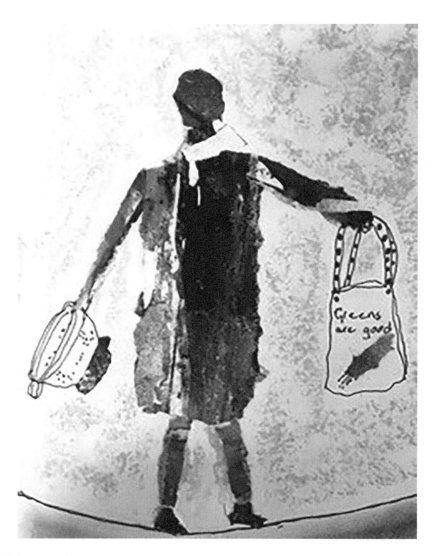

Tightrope walk

The 'melting pot'

One of my teachers, I can't remember now who it was, used to talk about diversity in food terms. We could think of using the different flavour and texture of what each of us brings to make soup. Or else we could use them to make a salad. The difference between those two dishes is that, in a soup, everything becomes more alike, uniting to offer a wholesome mix, within which each mouthful is almost the same. By contrast, in a salad, it is the contrast of flavours and textures that provide the interest. Every mouthful can be different.

Which is better? I think we need both. As a society, we need to acknowledge and accommodate our difference, and perhaps also begin to integrate it in a carefully chosen and considered variety of ways, always remembering that, for all species, diversity is necessary for survival:

- Some differences, like gender, have seemed like a given. Each of us is either M or F and this determines the direction and possibilities of our lives. Gender seems to be becoming more fluid now, with gender reassignment being frequently discussed in the media, and people feeling increasingly able to explore their gender identity more freely. Certainly, this has been the case in my client work.
- Other differences, like race, can blend over time. As more of us move or travel to different countries, children are born having a mixed cultural heritage. This brings its own challenges too (Eddo-Lodge, 2018).
- Sexuality is a difference that is not predictable, and often not obvious to other people at first, although we may think we know . . . Same sex marriage and the structural and societal benefits the institution of marriage brings may make any differences less conspicuous over time. Anyway, the younger people I meet often have a more fluid attitude to their sexuality.
- Some physical and mental 'impairments' are also not immediately obvious, while others are. I'm hesitating to give examples here because each of us has our own attitudes to our experience, and it's probably not helpful to have it labelled as a 'problem' by someone else. I know that several years ago, when I had to use a walking-stick for a time, I was shocked by how differently I was treated in public places. I remember being ignored sometimes by shop assistants and, in the street, having people either push past me or extravagantly (and to my mind patronizingly) gesturing for me to take priority.
- I am beginning to notice some differences that come with age too, like being called 'My Love' by shop assistants and bus drivers.

Variety is positive, but the problem with people being different is that some groups have more power, entitlement or resources than others. That power differential is something we need to be sensitive to as we work with others, I believe.

In writing this section, I will avoid the convention that takes a white, heterosexual, able-bodied male as some kind of 'standard' from which the rest of us deviate. This is because I don't want to bolster that as an attitude and, anyway, it's

outdated. I am writing from the point of view of my own experience and identity –
I can do no other. I know that yours is different. Despite our differences, I hope
we can find a place to meet. If I offend you because of my different attitudes and
experience, it is unintentional, something I have tried very hard to avoid, and
I hope you will feel able to forgive.

Race and ethnicity

The killing of George Floyd in Minneapolis in May 2020 brought the issue of
race and colour violently to the forefront, not for the first time but with seemingly
stronger emphasis. Black Lives Matter was the call that resulted in concerted
action from people of colour in response.

Symbols of the slave trade became targets. In Bristol, which is the nearest big
city, just across the Severn Bridge from where I live and very familiar to me, the
statue of slave trader Edward Colston was toppled and thrown into the harbour
in June of that year. This was only one of many attempts to re-contextualize the
building of privilege, wealth and empire that has taken place over centuries at the
expense of particular groups of people. The slave trade involved black people
being taken from their own countries to other parts of the world to work for the
benefit of white people and for no reward to themselves. This trade continued for
300 years (Eddo-Lodge, 2018). To aggrandize the perpetrators of that outrage
seems shocking and offensive, so I can understand why their monuments have
become targets. The fact that the slave trade was directly connected with food,
particularly sugar, makes discussion of it very relevant for this book.

I am white. This means I have privilege because of the history of the UK and
other colonial countries. As part of this history, some groups of people were
exploited in order to benefit others. I am one of the beneficiaries. **The standard
of living I enjoy now can be traced back to the prosperity created in Britain
by the exploitation of black slaves in the past.**

Sometimes I find it more difficult to focus on my privilege than it is to connect
with the injustice I feel as a woman from a working-class background, and I have
to be careful. I'm not so well off in comparison with many others. I do not have
access to the kind of privileges they enjoy. I do not have the power to exercise
my will in the way some others can. Are there hierarchies of injustice? If there
are, how helpful is it to try and identify who has suffered most? Nevertheless,
while I may feel that I am treated unjustly every day, **I have never been a slave,
neither has anyone in the history of my family, as far as I know**. It is important
to acknowledge the significance of my own feelings of injustice even if, in the
scheme of things, it is relatively minor because, if I cannot hold my own experience alongside that of others, I may feel injured and resentful, which may result in
backlash against any attempts at progress. This kind of backlash is already evident
very clearly in society at the moment.

In her 2009 book 'Being White in the Helping Professions', Judy Ryde suggests a way of approaching these seemingly irreconcilable points of view. She
focuses on the difference between non-dual thinking and dualistic thinking. A non-
dual approach permits us to acknowledge the fundamental 'truth' of each facet of

a situation, without attempting to come down on the side of either being right or wrong, better or worse. This kind of thinking is found in some spiritual traditions, and also in Gestalt, where it helps us understand the co-emergent nature of the relationship between person and world. Incidentally, Ryde observes that it was dualistic thinking that 'allowed the west to proceed with the project of colonization which is justified by seeing the colonized as an inferior type of human being' (2009, p. 115).

A few years ago, I did an arts-related course that was facilitated by a black man. All of the other participants were white too, and about equally split between women and men. The people were mostly professional and well-educated. Part of the introductory process in the group involved our being asked to identify and name the characteristics that people would notice about us as individuals when they first saw us. We had quite a long and challenging discussion between us, encompassing age, weight, neurodiversity and physical impairment. One thing was not mentioned. The facilitator himself had to prompt us. I decided to speak it. 'You're black'. I said, 'I don't come on many courses where the facilitator is black'. Almost immediately another group member said, 'I'm colour blind'. There was a buzz of approval at this statement and, while I felt uneasy about the potential risks of that position, it didn't feel like the time or place to prolong the discussion so, rightly or wrongly, I let the subject drop. I also felt like I was being invited to a place of shame for having mentioned something that shouldn't be talked about and I had to work hard not to go there. In my own defence, part of my thinking was about waiting to see how the facilitator himself responded and take a cue from that. In the end, the discussion sort of got dropped.

In her book 'Why I'm No Longer Talking to White People about Race' (2018, p. x), Reni Eddo-Lodge observes: 'The journey towards understanding structural racism still requires people of colour to prioritise white feelings'. How does this dynamic play out if there is a difference of race between practitioner and client? Actually, it's probably also important to note if there is no difference, depending on the context in which the meeting takes place. A sense of being the same or different from someone else is powerful and I return to this later.

Both Eddo-Lodge and Ryde suggest that some awareness training for white people in the history of colonialism and the privileges that come with being white might contribute towards finding a way to start redressing the injustice.

Colonialism

Is colonialism a thing of the past? If colonialism is defined as being a situation where a powerful incomer arrives and starts appropriating the resources of the current inhabitants, then it clearly is not. The Guardian ran an article on 2nd January 2021, which was written by their South-east Asia correspondent, Rebecca Ratcliffe. A community in Cambodia is claiming legal redress for having had their lands seized from them and used to produce sugar. Tate and Lyle, a major international sugar producer, was mentioned as having been involved. The report describes how, having been stripped of the means to grow their food, the community had to work for the sugar producer for low wages. This is so reminiscent of the situation following enclosure in eighteenth-century Britain, and here we are in the twenty-first century and it still seems acceptable for powerful vested interests to just take what they want. The Cambodian villagers are still fighting for justice and I will follow the progress of their claim for redress with interest.

At the same time, ordinary people in the west want cheap sugar. For myself, I would be very happy to pay extra for my sugar so that people in far-away countries are not exploited. Then I can afford it, and I try not to eat too much sugar anyway, for reasons that have been described very fully earlier on in the book. Many people are unable to pay more. Others are unwilling to do so. Our actions as individuals and families may seem tiny, but they lead to consequences that we may or may not want to acknowledge.

Gender

I'm starting this section with 'FIFI' – 'Fat is a Feminist Issue', the book by Susie Orbach. Its svelte presence in my bookcase has accompanied me through many life changes and house moves. When I took it down to write this section, I checked the date of its publication – 1988 – not, actually, as old as I thought, but still pretty old. . . . The language and approach took me back to another time, when 'women's lib' was a fresh and active movement. At that time, the 'pill' and other methods of contraception, plus the availability of pregnancy termination, had allowed women more freedom of choice around relationships, sex and motherhood. In the UK, the grammar school system and grants, which meant that the state paid for people to go to university, had made higher education more inclusive. The Equal Pay Act of 1970 had dispensed with there being two pay scales for jobs, one for males and another (substantially less) for females. Women could have bank accounts and mortgages in their own name. A state pension became available to women at age 60. For men, pension age was 65.

FIFI is a book about compulsive eating. It is also about women's experience in the world. – the toll it takes on a human being to be under constant pressure to look a certain way in order to be attractive to men and, at the same time, to provide care and nurture for others. It is a book about fear – the danger of what might happen to a person's sense of self as a consequence of attempting to comply with all these expectations. . . . When I first read it in the 1980s, I tried to allow myself to be aware of why I was afraid to be thin, but I didn't get very far. I was married, with a child and a job, and also a hunger to know and experience more of the world and to understand better what to make of it all. . . . I still have that hunger, but my relationship with the world and with food has changed enough for me to stay relatively thin. I lost weight 10 years ago, but I'm still getting used to how the world treats me differently. People stand too close to me, especially men. It's as though being fat gave me power over who could come close. Being smaller now puts me at the disposal of others. One time I was out shopping alone. Standing in the queue at the supermarket, I suddenly felt hands at my waist, pushing me out of the way. I turned around, and there was a man of around my own age, confidently at ease, 'I just wanted to get a newspaper'. He explained, pointing to where they were stacked on the shelf opposite, as though shifting me out of the way was perfectly justifiable. I felt alarmed and outraged. I felt like shouting and screaming at him for daring to treat me in that offhand way, but I knew the other people in the shop wouldn't get it and think me hysterical. So, I very coldly stood back, indicated the newspapers and said 'OK. But you're not allowed to touch me'. He did look a bit abashed then.

The big, strong people go out to hunt. They are more important, so they take more privileges than the smaller, weaker people who stay at home to take care of everything. Simone de Beauvoir was scathing about this hunter-gatherer mentality,

> men have always kept in their hands all concrete powers; since the early days of the patriarchy they have thought it best to keep woman in a state of dependence; their codes of law had been set up against her; and thus she has been definitely established as the Other.
>
> (1997, p. 171)

Here again the importance of the theme of difference, or otherness, is recognized as underlying the justification of oppression. The legacy from this primitive past means that women do the cooking, except for on special, ceremonial occasions, when men take on the task. Like at restaurants today, when top chefs are mostly men. There are many men who are 'celebrity chefs' too. In this role, people like Jamie Oliver and Nigel Slater focus on the domestic sphere, even though that is traditionally women's place. They celebrate the delight of a home-cooked meal and togetherness.

Nigella Lawson evokes domesticity by observing, 'I'm not saying the kitchen is always necessarily a zen place to be, but it can be a safe place for the frenetic soul' (2020, p. vii). It is meaningful and satisfying to prepare a meal for family and friends. It feels like an honour to nurture those we love and watch them thrive. It is also dangerous, because, crucial though it is to human development and well-being, it is low status, so being involved with these acts risks lack of esteem, recognition and reward, unless you happen to be one of the few who are famous.

Equal pay and equal access to work have meant that, for a couple, both partners need to work to earn enough money to bring up a family. It is no longer easily afford-able for wives to stay at home to look after children, as was the case for a lot of families (although not mine) when I was a child. Despite all the time that has passed since the Equal Pay Act, survey after survey shows that women earn less than men as their careers develop, because women still carry the main responsibility for child-care. One thing that has equalled up is the pension age. Women who for most of their lives expected to be able to retire at 60 had to wait until 62, then 65, then 67. So now, many men in well-paid jobs retire close to age 50 with generous occupational pensions, while women have to keep on working because they do not have access to such pensions. Their career pattern has had to accommodate time away from paid work to undertake (unpaid) caring responsibilities for their children, so there was less opportunity to accrue one. Many of these same women are now caring for frail par-ents as well as continuing to earn a living. I know mine is only one point of view, and that there are many others, but mine is one that shows me a disparity between what men can have and what women can have that I see echoed in many other situations.

Food is a symbol of how society works. Many families where both parents have jobs outsource cooking to supermarket ready-meals or take-aways. Earlier chapters in this book have discussed how processed food and high contents of refined sugar and fat lead to what we now call 'lifestyle' diseases. Maybe the crisis we are experiencing will encourage us to re-think our priorities, re-balancing how we define 'value' and rewarding caring that involves access to healthy foodstuffs and healthy meals for all of us, including but not exclusively that done by women. Perhaps recognizing the true value of caring for one another may make it more attractive to both men and women.

Class (opportunity)

At the risk of seeming to prioritize men's feelings, in the same way Eddo-Lodge identifies that people of colour have to do for white people, for the sake of fairness and inclusivity, it is important to recognize that many men feel disadvantaged too. Inequality is a fundamental characteristic of our society, as I discussed in the previous chapter. In both the UK and the USA, some parts of the country are more affluent than others. Here in the UK, London is where the resources are, and where a lot of the whole country's resources go. Until recently, the political view was that investing in London, reinforcing its place as a world city, would trickle down affluence into the rest of the country. This reminds me of the belief that has formed part of capitalist economic theory, that entrepreneurs should be helped to make a lot of money because it would trickle down to everyone else. I think both of these beliefs have been recognized as being false now, although they have been given a generous opportunity to work, maybe too much of an opportunity. Perhaps the lack of a viable alternative made a different approach seem unachievable. This has changed now, as we will see in the next chapter.

Meanwhile, young people who cannot access the well-paid professions because of the relative scarcity of those kinds of jobs, or lack of education, or inability to belong to the right networks, are working in bars or coffee-shops on zero-hours contracts. Even some highly educated, hard-working professionals, like teachers, frequently have only yearly contracts as their security of employment. When they are in secure, reasonably paid jobs, men have now to compete with women for advancement. They may be concerned that the legislation and procedures that protect women's opportunities will be detrimental for their own. In some situations, they may be right, in others definitely not. It is almost certainly the case that re-balancing the privileges enjoyed by men and white people will mean that we all have to give up some of our advantages for the benefit of the whole. It takes insight and maturity to be able to do that. A sense of there being enough to go round, and trust in the societal structure, is essential too. So how can we begin to build that kind of environment? I return to this later in the chapter.

Ability and disability

The focus of the book is food and mental health, so in this section I want mainly to discuss the conditions, both mental and physical, that are linked with diet. The connection between food and the development and health of the brain is now well documented. We have seen a rise over recent years in the numbers of children born with autism that has been connected with modern food habits and also with increased levels of pollution (Korn, 2016). There has also been an increase in Alzheimer's and other diseases of dementia in older adults. Dementia is linked with inflammation, the body's immune response both to harmful substances within the body and to damage suffered as a result of harm from outside the body (cuts, burns, grazes, . . .). The body reacts to refined carbohydrates and artificial trans fats (like hydrogenated vegetable fats) found in processed foods and also to alcohol with an inflammatory response (Korn, 2016). The effects of poor diet on mental health seem to be particularly noticeable at the beginning and end of our lives, when the gut microbiome is more vulnerable (Mayer, 2016).

I will talk about age-related dementia in the next section. But first, some good news, despite this recognition of the quite shocking effects of our present diet and lifestyle. Neurodiversity is becoming more accepted in the public sphere, and the attributes that accompany it are being appreciated. The nature presenter Chris Packham is open about his Asperger's diagnosis, so is activist Greta Thunberg. Seeing how impressive they are and how much they have achieved is likely to be a contributing factor to more general acceptance of the condition.

Depression is a very common mental health condition that has links with diet. It is also connected with long-term stress (Korn, 2016). Dietary deficits connected with depression include omega-3 fatty acids (found in oily fish and walnuts) and B and C vitamins (from fresh fruit and vegetables). A deficit in the trace element magnesium has also been identified in connection with depression (Korn, 2016). Magnesium used to come from the soil, but there is less of it available now because of the modern farming techniques I have discussed in the previous chapter. Some people (including me) take magnesium (Epsom salts) baths as a remedy.

Strangely, it is harder for me to talk about the physical disability that comes with being overweight. Maybe because it is closer to home. I notice the effects of many years of carrying too much weight on my own body, my joints, particularly in the lower part of my body have become worn, affecting the way I can move around in the world. As I walk about in the streets, I notice people who are overweight, and how they seem to me to be restricted and effortful in their movements. I don't know whether these individuals experience disability, and it is not for me to decide. The decision I can and have made is not to let my own issues become disabling. To that end, I work hard at various forms of physical exercise.

Other 'lifestyle' diseases that affect the physical body include type 2 diabetes, heart disease, stroke, irritable bowel syndrome, arthritis and asthma. Poor diet and stress together seem to have a contributory role in the emotional and physical impact of our current lifestyles. Both physical and mental issues will have an effect on mental health and wellbeing because, again, we are whole beings and not a random gathering of disconnected parts.

Age

If there is a recurring theme in this book, it is the importance of a diet that is rich in vegetables and fruit, contains proteins, fats and oils, and complex carbohydrates (potatoes in their skins, brown rice, wholemeal bread). Avoiding refined sugar, trans fats and an excess of alcohol is also important. Our diet and lifestyle can catch up with us as we age, but the good news is that changing our habits can help, even at that time. Contributing factors to mental and physical health as we age include:

- Diet
- Exercise for the body (especially aerobic exercise like brisk walking)
- Exercise for the mind: creative pursuits, hobbies, puzzles, new experiences, different challenges
- Exercise for the emotions – express yourself and connect with others at deeper levels
- Be vigilant in noticing if watching television stops being entertainment and starts becoming a way of passing the time, or a distraction from everyday realities
- Control blood pressure
- Spend time with people and in social situations
- Avoid or address stress, anxiety and depression
- Sleep well

(Leyse-Wallace, 2008)

For those who are very far away from experiencing any of the challenges of ageing, I would like to assure you that, despite any physical changes, we remain human beings as we get older. 'The elderly' (I hate that term) are not a separate species. I don't quite know why conversations across age groups follow the pattern they sometimes do of the younger person speaking loudly and slowly, and with exaggerated care, and the older person talking about their age and ailments. When I overhear that kind of conversation, it feels like both parties fall into a ritual form of how they think they 'should' communicate. Maybe I will gain some insight about that as I become older myself.

Sexuality and transgender

I found the 'Alice B. Toklas Cook Book' on-line, although, for some time in its life, it had been in a second-hand bookshop. I could tell by the pencil markings on the first page. I knew her from her 'Autobiography', the one her life-partner, Gertrude Stein, had written for her. In their writings, they tend to refer to one another using their full names, so I will do the same. Gertrude Stein wrote experimental books, poetry and plays and Alice B. Toklas wrote cookbooks – and cooked food. The two American women lived together in Paris in the early twentieth century and knew everybody. Lunch for Picasso was fish – bass, decorated with two shades of mayonnaise, hard-boiled eggs with truffles and 'chopped *fines-herbes*' (1983, p. 30). Picasso approved of the dish but wondered if it might not have been more suitable for Matisse, who was also a visitor (a bit of an in-joke, referring to Matisse's style of painting and choice of colour).

Life for the two women was not all about gallery openings and lunch parties. They had to evacuate Paris twice, on account of both the First and Second World Wars. Alice B. Toklas was already familiar with emergencies, having been caught up in the San Francisco earthquake and fire of 1906. On the aftermath of that she observes, 'I had been able to secure two hams and my father had brought back two hundred cigarettes. With these one might, he said, not only exist but be able to be hospitable' (1983, p. 31). When the Second War sent them once again to the French countryside, securing provisions became a big part of their way of life. She observed that, 'it is not with money that one buys on the black market but with one's personality' (1983, p. 207). These two women had no shortage of personality and lived their lives with style and flair. Not all gay people have such style and flair, but the stereotype has some truth to it, in my experience. I won-der if this attitude is a consequence of the potential precariousness of a lifestyle that has not always been accepted by society. Maybe sociability and investing in making everyday encounters with others rewarding for them is a way of making difference more acceptable. Perhaps emphasizing difference through flamboyant appearance or behaviour is another way of coming to terms with it.

In a same-sex couple, both 'hunting' and 'caring' may be more equally shared among the partners. Alice B. Toklas certainly took the role of 'forethoughtful housekeeper' (1983, p. 31), while Gertrude Stein drove the car and tended to the hedges, but there was a tender equality between them that I have seen in other same-sex relationships, of either sex. Same-sex couples have mainly been child-less, but that is changing now, as both methods of conception and attitudes evolve. Caring for children may change this dynamic.

I like to think that each of us carries the potential for both hunting and caring. I also notice that gender characteristics, whether innate or developed in response to environmental influences, find a balance somewhere. When people decide to change their biological and/or social gender, this balance seems to need to be rene-gotiated by the individual involved and also by the people around them. I would like to be able to transcend gender stereotypes, but I notice how deeply ingrained they are in my body and psyche, resulting in attitudes that I need to be very careful to bring into my awareness and ponder. I recognize in myself the desire to be able to consume like a man, although I have the body of a woman and society treats me like one, and this is a conflict for me.

Language

Another privilege I feel I possess is that of having English as a first language. I only became aware of the significance of it when I started hanging out in work environments with Italians mainly, but other Europeans too. English is the default common language in Europe and, I think, throughout the world. I have noticed this particularly while travelling. A quarrel between a Frenchman and a Scandi-navian on the High-Speed Train from Paris to Turin was conducted in English. Eventually the Scandinavian won, and I think the outcome was just because the Frenchman previously wouldn't move his seat to let the Scandinavian's wife and child sit down.

International English is different from that spoken by those of us who have it as a first language. This is not to say that the English spoken by Americans and

Australians is the same as that spoken by Brits. I think we would save ourselves a lot of confusion if we understood clearly that Americans and Brits speak very different languages from one another, even though a lot of the words are the same.

I try not to take advantage of my language privilege and I use the French I learned at school and the Italian I began to study a few years ago as best I can. This brings me to the reason I have chosen to include a section on language among this discussion of difference and diversity. Language is connected with how we express ourselves in the world and consequently with how others perceive us. The possibilities open to us for relating with others are deeply connected with verbal communication. I used to take it very much for granted that I could express my feelings and ideas with others, and also have a multi-levelled awareness of what they were communicating with me, both spoken and unspoken. I was proud of my ability to pick up and respond to nuances of the communication on both sides, and my professional training was all about honing the skills needed to be able to do that. I use these highly developed faculties in different ways, according to the situation. I might comfort or encourage a family member or friend, reflect a potentially valuable insight back to a client or use my skills to win an argument or resolve a problem in a more public domain. The way I speak, my accent and into-nation, communicates a lot about me in terms of my background, education, life-style and disposable income, although perhaps not all these signals are received completely identically by every listener because each one will have their own way of interpreting what I say depending on their background and experience. I reveal my intelligence and authority in what I say, which is crucial in my line of work, but also necessary for negotiating any unfamiliar situation or new environment

When I speak in a foreign language in a strange place, all those advantages become unavailable to me and I lose status because of it. In tourist situations, this is somehow more manageable, because it is expected that visitors will not speak the language of the country, so other factors come into play particularly national-ity, in my experience. I notice that being a Brit (and obviously western) seems to give me a subtle advantage over people from some parts of the world, but not from others, and it is interesting to notice which nationalities are accorded status and privilege at a particular time. Confidence and demeanour also play a part in how 'strangers' are assessed. Because of this I have learned now that, if I want to complain about something in a hotel, or in another tourist-related situation I do so in English because it gives me an advantage.

Away from the places tourists go, language takes on a different significance. I have been in situations in work contexts in Italy where everyone else is Ital-ian, many of the other people know each other from a shared connection with a particular organization, and the majority of them are unable or prefer not to speak any English. The English-speaking Italian friends who have introduced me into the situation have occasionally been stared at in alarm as I started to try out the Italian I had begun to learn! Even though my Italian has improved now, I know that I cannot express myself fully and gracefully, nuances (and sometimes whole sentences) are lost on me, and that this affects my ease, competence and authority. I have to work hard in other ways to overcome that as best I can.

Visitors, and particularly immigrants whose language skills are limited, are unable to reveal their full identities to the existing inhabitants of their new host country. I believe this is why for non-first-language speakers, learning English is such a crucial skill, whether they are travelling to the UK or to other parts of the world. Speaking English gives access to communication internationally. It seems important to me that those of us who have it as a first language do not take our privilege for granted.

Maybe this is something personal to me, but I miss having command of the language when I speak one in which I am not fluent. It has seemed to me that in some situations I have been dismissed as seeming stupid because my communication is so limited. Because of this, I would like to suggest here that lack of proficiency in a language does not mean someone is stupid, only that they are still learning.

A shift in consciousness?

What does it mean for us to be the 'other'? Generally, we have a deep sense of where we belong, and are uncomfortably sensitive to situations in which we step outside of what we know and perceive ourselves as being different. Why are human beings, so acutely aware of when people are like us and when they are not like us?

I wouldn't even have thought to frame such a question until I went to Budapest in 2019. It was for a conference, organized by the European Association for Gestalt Therapy, although it was attended by Gestaltists from many other parts of the world too. One of the keynote speeches was made by Gordon Wheeler. He is an American, and among the foremost Gestalt writers and thinkers in English. In his speech (Wheeler, 2019), he gave an account of the development of the human species, beginning with our life in the trees. He explained how one of our deeply embedded characteristics is to react to risk by strengthening an attitude of 'us and them': identifying the group with which we feel we belong and demonizing those outside it. In other words, favouring people like us and rejecting people that are not like us. For me, this was a revelation. I had seen this kind of dynamic unfolding daily in news bulletins. The 'America First' policy of the then president Trump, attitudes to immigration all over Europe, including in the UK, the decision for Britain to break from the European Union.

I notice it also in myself. I find it easier to ask for directions from a woman my own age when lost in a strange place, whatever country I'm in. I fondly remember the very courteous Parisienne I encountered in Le Marais, who replied in French to my enquiry about the nearest Metro station, even though it was obvious I was a visitor, and her English was probably way better than my French. Also, the lady in Palermo who went to great lengths to find out the location of my B&B. She and her friends chatted in a very friendly way to me in Italian, once we had found the place and were outside the door. Somehow, it seems to me, finding a commonality, even where there is a lot of difference, helps, which is probably why the Gestalt practitioners from all over the world found common ground in Budapest. We have a shared interest and language – the language of Gestalt.

There are other situations when my fear of difference (and I do recognize it as fear at certain times) leads to potentially more threatening outcomes. I notice that in a public place, if someone is speaking loudly on a mobile phone, I feel annoyed. If that person is speaking loudly in a different language, I feel even more annoyed. The feeling goes something like, 'This is my home ground. You are the stranger here, you need to defer to me and make an effort to be like me, stop annoying me. . .'. I didn't like this reaction in myself, but there didn't seem to be much I could do about it, apart from being very careful not to act on it. Wheeler's ideas helped me understand why I feel this way, and also why it is so difficult **not** to feel like it, after thousands of years of evolution.

One of the very few Greek words I know is philoxenia, which means love of the stranger, the desire to be hospitable. I have heard ancient stories of travellers in remote areas of every part of the world, not only in Greece or other parts of Europe, who have had to rely on this hospitality. When there are no Travelodges, no hostels for backpackers and no room at the inn, it is the only option, and both locals and travellers seem to take their responsibilities to one another very seriously. In return for food and shelter, the traveller tells her or his story. This traditional exchange is a currency that goes back time out of mind. . . . Though, even today, when I stay in the homes of friends, I notice they expect the tale of my journey, or of the places I have been to before arriving with them, and I always have something ready that I hope will be interesting. Writing this, I wonder if they are aware as they listen that they will form part of the story I tell in the next place I arrive at, whether it is in a new country or on the pages of a new piece of writing.

Although we have developed traditions for recognizing the wariness we have of the unfamiliar 'other' and rituals for addressing any unease, Wheeler suggested that human beings may need at this stage of our evolution to move on from it. He talks about the possibility of our undergoing a collective shift in consciousness in order to overcome this primitive (though historically useful) characteristic. Gestaltists do not normally speak of shifts in consciousness, and, while I was convinced by the need for it to happen, I was completely baffled about how to accomplish it or even what was actually meant by the term! As a consequence, when I arrived back home from Budapest, I had a lot of research on the subject ahead of me, the outcomes of which I describe in the next section.

If you want to listen to Gordon's speech for yourself, it is available on YouTube and there is a link to it in the 'Resources' section towards the end of the book.

Models of 'consciousness'

After quite a lot of reading, I understood that nobody really knows what consciousness is (Burkeman, 2015). Scientists and philosophers are still speculating about the nature of consciousness and what having it means for us as human beings and for the world we inhabit. Yet the lived reality for all of us is that we do have a sense of being a discrete identity, separate from our environments while deeply interconnected with them (this may be beginning to sound familiar from Chapter 4). I understand that I am conscious (have consciousness?) even though I might not completely understand the nature and implications of it. I have also experienced episodes in my life that feel like shifts in consciousness, usually connected with periods of significant change, like finally taking myself out of a job where I was deeply unhappy, after years of finding it impossible to make the move.

Despite discovering the limitations of current understanding, I persisted in my quest, hoping to reveal something about consciousness that I would find meaningful. I firmly believed that, if I understood more, it would help me identify the possibilities available to us as a species as we tackle the existential challenges we face. So, I read on, and also started some conversations with friends who know more than I about the topic of consciousness. In this way, I found Ken Wilber. In his book 'Integral Spirituality' (2006), he had plenty to say about consciousness, much of which illuminated the kind of shift in consciousness that Wheeler seemed to be recommending. Wilber emphasizes the distinction between states of consciousness (waking, sleeping, dreaming in some well-known systems) and levels of consciousness. It is possible to move between the levels of consciousness as he defines them, and there is definitely a hierarchy of progression. The levels of consciousness Wilber identifies are:

1   Egocentric, I care about myself.
2   Ethnocentric, I care about people who are close and connected with me.
3   Worldcentric, I care about everybody and everything.

With these three, Wilber included a fourth level, from the work of feminist author Carol Gilligan. In her book 'In a Different Voice' (1982), Gilligan identified a subsequent stage of 'integration', at which level it is possible for people to incorporate the characteristics of the other gender. Wilber (2006, p. 12) defined 'feminine' characteristics as being concerned with 'relationship, care and responsibility' and 'masculine' characteristics as prioritizing 'autonomy, justice and rights'. Integration, then, would look like the ability to access all these potentials and use them to best effect in any situation.

While I know I am nowhere near the end of my own journey, either in life generally or in my understanding of consciousness, I have identified a potential direction of travel. I think I have moved on from a completely Egocentric stance, to come to what seems like an Ethnocentric point of view. I notice difference and try to neutralize it somehow, for example, when I chose to ask directions from the women in Paris and Sicily. Alternatively, I can remind myself of my own struggles with language, when I become irritated by hearing someone speaking in a foreign language loudly on their mobile phone nearby. Eventually, I hope developing a Worldcentric attitude may help me emphasize the many ways in which I am the same as every other human being, rather than tending to highlight the ways in which I am different. This awareness may then enable me finally to become able to transcend the gender binary and integrate the autonomy, justice and rights potential for interaction more fully with the relationship, care and responsibility aspects connected directly (by Wilber and Gilligan) with my gender.

This may be something like the kind of shift of consciousness Wheeler thinks we need in order to address the structural inequalities that seem inherent in the doings of humanity. Those inequalities continue to allow it to be the case that some of us enjoy privileges at the expense of others. If enough of us became more alive to our shared experience of being human, it would be more difficult to tolerate the kind of inequalities I described earlier in the chapter. Yet I know that diversity is essential if any species is to flourish. I also know how important difference is for creativity and in joint problem solving. So, the issue is more subtle than attempting to replace alienation with identification, and my search had not ended.

For me, there was still something missing from Wilber's way of conceptualizing experience.

I felt dissatisfied with the way he talked about consciousness with a focus only on the individual. In Chapter 4, I explored the metaphor of the 'contact boundary', an imaginary seam that both connects us to the environment and keeps us separate from it. The dynamic here is one of a mutual, responsive exchange. Change is initiated not only by an individual acting autonomously, but also by a collective momentum coming from the environment.

In my day-to-day experience, I recognize that sometimes I am initiating change, and sometimes I am responding to environmental forces and undercurrents that require me to change. Yet the process is so subtly responsive that it is difficult to know where the impulse arises, whether it is from me or from my environment. Attempting to pinpoint one or the other as a definite source is probably useless, and not helpful anyway for understanding and responding to what is unfolding at the contact boundary. And here I am, back with the foundation principles of Gestalt.

Returning to the book 'Gestalt Therapy' (Perls, Hefferline and Goodman, 1992 [1951]), I find the assertion that 'contacting occurs at the surface-boundary *in* (italics in original) the field organism/environment' (p. 258) and 'the contact boundary is so to speak, the specific organ of awareness of the novel situation of the field' (p. 259). Individuals and their social environments evolve in different ways, but the permeability of the boundary allows awareness to flow between. I notice that my increased understanding of the importance of certain foods is changing how I speak and act in my day-to-day activities. I have also noticed that other people have been affected by my choices and have changed their own buying habits.

The ground of experience laid down by individuals and societies is where something that can be recognized as consciousness may be situated. Fortunately, it does evolve, and one of the catalysts for this progression is the response to environmental challenges. Here I include environmental both in the Gestalt sense – meaning challenges mainly initiated by my surroundings rather than by my self – and in the literal, everyday sense of the environment of the natural world, that of our home planet, our Earth. At this point, Gestalt language and everyday speech seem to coincide around the climate emergency.

I realize I have not pinned down what consciousness actually is and what it does. I believe humans find it difficult to separate from aspects of being that are so fundamental to our nature and, so far, we cannot achieve a perspective that helps us understand them fully. Consciousness is one of these mysteries that might need to be contemplated with awe rather than contained by a rigid definition. I believe the relationship of humans with our environment is similarly ineffable: it is so much part of our nature that we cannot distance ourselves from it enough to perceive it clearly. This, for me, is how we came to let the climate catastrophe happen.

Does this mean that there is an environmental consciousness as well as millions of personal consciousnesses? My own view is that I think there may actually be something resembling that. One of the approaches that seeks to understand and explore this kind of collective sentience is Field Theory.

Field Theory

In this context I want to discuss Field Theory as it was developed by Kurt Lewin, a psychologist who was born in Germany, but lived and worked in the USA in the middle of the twentieth century. Much of our current understanding of group and organizational dynamics is influenced by his work. See:

https://en.wikipedia.org/wiki/Kurt_Lewin

for more information.

We often hear of Quantum Field Theory these days, following the discoveries of physicists working in this area. Although I imagine that at some level quantum and Lewinian theories reflect one another, that discussion is not for here, because this is a practical rather than a theoretical book. Coincidentally, though, Lewin is credited with having coined the phrase 'There is nothing as practical as a good theory'. For the context see:

https://journals.sagepub.com/doi/pdf/10.1177/1534484305276176.

Field Theory is rich and, for me, sometimes complex and indigestible, so here I will examine how its application can be useful to a practitioner in the field of health. Lewin's proposition was that individuals cannot really be understood except in relation to their environment. We have been exploring this connection over several chapters, so it is likely to be a familiar concept. Lewin situates our experience of being at the contact boundary within a dynamic field that can both influence and be influenced by all the interactions taking place within its sphere. Lewin sometimes referred to the fields in which we are all personally embedded as 'life space' and that seems to me like a simple and direct way of describing and understanding them.

See www.britannica.com/science/life-space for more information.

The people with whom we work enter our life space bringing their own life space with them and are connected to us through the dynamics of the field we co-inhabit (Nevis, 1987). Consequently, it may be helpful to know some characteristics of the way fields function in order to understand their nature more fully and recognize the possibilities and limitations inherent within them. Those whose role is specifically concerned with how effectively a field is organizing, like managers, organizational consultants, HR and other communications specialists, for example, may also be interested in how to facilitate some change or learning within their own particular field according to this model, if it is not already familiar.

One of the most respected commentators on Field Theory in the Gestalt world is Malcolm Parlett. I have referred extensively to his work in writing this section

(Parlett, 1991), although any inaccuracies and misunderstandings within it are entirely my own.

1 Meaning comes from the whole picture

Everything in a field is connected to every other aspect and we can only make sense of what is happening by comprehending the whole. Like the composition of the Monalisa discussed in Chapter 4, in which the figure and her background together are what makes the smile both mysterious and meaningful for the viewer. The smile is how we define her, but the placement of her hands, the neckline of her dress, the line of trees behind and everything else that da Vinci chose to include in the painting all contribute to our sense of wholeness and satisfaction and so allow ourselves to be captured by what she portrays. Of course, a portrait is not the equivalent of an alive, dynamic human life space, although we, as observers, might perceive her differently according to how our own life spaces are currently configuring. The relational field between two or more humans is influenced by all the factors present in it.

Case example 1

Here is an example of how this principle might be applied professionally in an everyday situation. After working so hard on a tricky-to-reach root-canal filling, a specialist dentist might be surprised at how angry his patient was that he had drilled away a tiny area of an adjacent canine tooth in order to facilitate access. He knew he would be able to restore the tooth very easily at the follow-up visit. What he did not know was that she was going on holiday the next day and that the chipped tooth mattered because it was a very special holiday, and she would be meeting significant new people. He didn't know because he hadn't asked, assuming the patient would see things the same way he did, yet she had brought her own life-space into their shared field, and her response was in tune with that.

Case example 2

Josh was preparing for university after being successful in his exams. His family sent him to their local surgery because they could not understand why he had suddenly become worried about his appearance and anxious about his food intake. His GP, Allen, had known him from a child and remembered him as being well-mannered and reasonably confident. He was surprised, then, when the young man arrived for his appointment, to notice that puberty had not been kind to him. There was a fierce rash on his chin, and he seemed underweight and apprehensive. Allen took the time to ask Josh how he felt about going to university and he replied very positively. They talked about Josh's eating patterns and he agreed to keep a food and mood diary and come back for another appointment in a month's time. Josh's father came with him to the next appointment. He was heartily dismissive when Allen tried to discuss the food and mood diary and said that his son would be fine when he arrived at university and started his course. After all, he (the father) had done exactly the same degree and it had 'been the making of him'. Josh told Allen that, indeed, he was just feeling a bit nervous about the big change he was soon to experience, that he was feeling better, and it would all turn out fine. Allen watched father and son leave his office and hoped Josh was right, although it seemed likelier that he might need more support and hoped he would be able to access it when he started at university. Seeing father and son together had revealed to Allen a lot more about the history and relational dynamic operating in the family (Josh's life space) exposing the possibilities and limitations for himself in his health professional role.

2   **Here and now**
A field only ever exists in the present. It cannot be recreated or revisited or, indeed, stay the same. Just like for us as individuals who are in moment-by-moment unfolding connection with our own particular environment (see Chapter 5), within a field each new 'now' is unique to the moment, although it is informed and tempered by what has gone before and carries the potential for how it may evolve. Now is really all that we can know. Our organs of perception: eyes, ears, nose, mouth, skin . . . only operate in the present. We orientate ourselves spontaneously in response to our sensory awareness, although sometimes what we perceive can be so powerful, or so unusual that we feel perturbed. We call this capacity our 'sixth sense', or intuition. Some practitioners, group facilitators, for example, deliberately cultivate this body-focused sensory awareness because it opens possibilities for new insights that can be shared with others who are directly involved in the field being explored. Of course, we also have the capacity to reprocess what we experience through memory, re-living the moment in our minds and re-experiencing our reactions. We also use the ability the mind has to imagine what might have happened, or what could still happen. . . . Each of these possibilities is valuable to us in our meaning making both individually and collectively yet, by then, the field has continued to constellate according to its own logic and a new moment has arrived. Significantly, our previous actions and reactions have contributed to the way this new now has taken shape.

3   **Field-based awareness**
In the same way that water finds its level, fields naturally organize themselves into the most favourable balance that is currently achievable (Nevis, 1987). This process unfolds in accordance with dynamics that may only become clearly understood by observing them. Discovering more about the various aspects of a field is the usual way of exploring our experience of it. This happens naturally as we negotiate our family and community interactions. The universal 'How are you?' is a basic version of it. In work environments, the enquiry can become more formal, ranging from a casual 'What happened when. . .' question to a Critical Incident investigation on a hospital ward. Sharing our experiences of being within them is how fields (and life spaces) can evolve and shift.

Fields for growing

Fields are complex, ever-changing and nebulous. They cannot be grasped and manipulated because they morph into something different at the attempt. So how is it at all possible to facilitate growth and change towards a particular goal as a field evolves? In this section, the focus will initially be on the field of work because that has direct relevance for us in our roles as health professionals. Later, wider, societal change will be explored because it forms part of the context within which our client work takes place and has an impact on it as a consequence.

Work

Practitioners often have particular, contracted roles in their work fields that go with their job titles. Sometimes a practitioner's responsibility is to work within a field by carrying out the activities for which the organization is responsible. Other practitioners work **with** a field, attending to how the organizational activities are being carried out and responsible for their being accomplished in optimal ways. Many roles may include both spheres. Organizations probably work better if all those involved give some attention to how the whole thing works, or how different parts of the organization work together when it is very large. Although, as with everything, balance is fundamental, the core activity or activities – what the organization was set up for – are paramount. Doing the 'wrong' thing really well does not make for good progress. Being able to identify activity that is central to an organization's core purpose means that effort can be directed most productively. Recognizing the distinction between the core activity and the action that is needed to make the organization operate optimally to deliver it, can support an organization's effectiveness (Cockman, Evans and Reynolds, 1992).

Formal structures that support how an organization is run include:

- Hierarchies, management, leadership, direction
- Support functions like HR, finance and procurement, cleaning and maintenance
- Policies and procedures
- Mission Statements

Informal elements that influence organizational coherence include:

- Meaningful boundaries
- Clear roles
- Informal hierarchies: experience, technical expertise, position, force of character. . .
- Appropriate rewards: money, recognition, job satisfaction, sense of belonging
- Recognition of the significance of the culture of the organization
- The collective emotional 'tone' which is often easy to pick up from being present in the organizational field. In some places it is strongly 'can do', in others 'we care' is the message that permeates the atmosphere, and there are many others. . .

Society

Reflecting on societal change, I can see how in my own lifetime the society in which I am embedded has been through a whole cycle. I have witnessed the resurgence of affluence after the bleak, frugal years following the war, the conspicuous consumption of the late twentieth century, and now the crisis of pollution, climate change and food production that challenges us.

During that time, a lot of ordinary people have become more affluent. We have been able to afford holidays abroad and consumer goods like cars and laptops. Eating out in restaurants became commonplace towards the end of the twentieth century, although, when I was a child, my family would never have been able to afford to eat in a restaurant. I remember visiting Bristol Zoo and seeing all the privileged people enjoying pots of tea and dainty sandwiches served on white tablecloths in the tea-rooms there. We had brought our own picnic over from Wales on the train with us and sat on the grass to eat it. I looked with envy through the tea-room window and felt excluded.

I enjoyed the possibility of going to cafés and restaurants when the world opened up to me as a teenager. I remember my first experience of eating at an Indian restaurant from when I was visiting ex-schoolfriends who were studying in London. My most vivid memory of the meal is of dipping a shard of poppadom into yoghurt and mint sauce. I had never seen a poppadom before, and I thought the mint sauce was one of the loveliest things I had ever tasted. My friends' college was just around the corner from Kensington High Street and department stores like Derry and Toms were still open then. But Biba's was there too and that was a revelation for a girl up from Wales. There was no Topshop or Next in British towns then, or any boutiques selling up-to-date fashion. There were some up-market department stores, but my clothes mostly came from the British Home Stores, which was a bit like a down-market Marks and Spencer's at the time, and which has since become extinct.

Now the local High Street is about to change again, with the rise of online shopping. We have become more conscious of the fallout of so-called 'cheap' fashion, on the environment and on the workers in the industry, whether they are in China or Leicester. Indian restaurants are commonplace, and it is possible to eat cuisines from many parts of the world within only a few miles travel from home. I am also aware that these are not really the cuisine of India or China, or even of Italy now, because I have travelled and read. I feel like I have seen the rise of a particular way of life and that, now, I am witnessing its decline. What we can afford financially, we can no longer afford in terms of wellbeing and, more crucially, we cannot continue to consume like this and also continue to exist.

What makes change? We know from Field Theory that fields are always changing, that you can never experience exactly the same configuration twice, and that every element of a field is a more or less significant contributor to the whole. The whole field is where we discover meaning. The meaning I made of my society evolved from the excitement of there being more possibilities available to me: tasting food from foreign countries, trying fashion that exploded the whole culture of wearing clothes, certainly in the west, and in other parts of the world too, where there was sufficient wealth. I have been able to afford financially to throw away clothes, shoes, houseware, ornaments and even books when my drawers and cupboards began to overflow with them. . . . I cringe as I write it now because I could never really afford to be so cavalier with the world's finite resources and the reckoning is here.

The meaning I make now of my society is that we have become bloated. Having access to just enough to be able to live a productive and satisfying life evolved into the expectation of constant growth – of always being able to have more. Equally worrying is that this is only true for some people, because the inequalities have also grown. Another new configuration needs to emerge. The political and economic systems that have supported this lifestyle also form part of this reconfiguration and I explore this further in the next chapter.

Difference, diversity and change

One thing that has changed for the better, in my opinion is the way people who are 'different' are perceived by society. More people are aware of racist and sexist language and behaviour and it is less generally acceptable than it was in the past, although in some contexts it still happens. I have heard several young men with whom I work talk about their not wanting to be 'pussy-whipped'. They tend to look uncomfortable then, maybe because of using the word in my presence but also, I would like to think, because they are aware of the sexism and potential misogyny identified with it and the consequences those attitudes have for society. The way we approach and resolve our individual differences reflects the civility of our society. There is no equivalent of the term 'pussy-whipped' to describe a situation where a woman has done what a man wants. Is it just me, or is there some unacknowledged assumption that this is how things should be? To reject the needs and wishes of someone important to you who is a woman because someone else might accuse you of being 'pussy-whipped' is distasteful and demeans everyone, in my opinion.

Same-sex marriage is possible now in the UK. This seemed inconceivable to me until very shortly before it came into law. When I was growing up, homosexual relationships were illegal for men and, if the topic ever did come up, there were remarks about its being impossible for women. I went to the wedding of two of my women friends and I noticed how the relatives who had also been invited smiled approvingly at same-sex couples in the room, even though they were in opposite-sex couples themselves. It surprised me a bit, and also gave me hope. It is also more common for same-sex couples to have children and I think this embeddedness in family structures will begin to change the attitude of society in general.

People with disabilities can no longer be excluded from public events because they might get in the way of other people in an emergency, something that regularly happened before disability legislation was adopted. There are limits to what has been achieved in all these areas, and backlashes and backsliding, but these measures can be seen as the primitive beginning of a movement towards Wilber's Worldcentric point of view, in which other people and beings matter, however unlike 'us' they are.

Reflecting on how the societal change I have experienced has come about, contextualizing it in the intimate exchange between an individual and their environment that takes place at the contact boundary, and also in the field dynamics that hold sway, I notice that we as individuals both influence and are influenced by society. While writing this book, I have changed my eating habits, so my shopping habits have also changed. Decisions about how any of us spends our money are powerful in this market-driven economy that has evolved to observe and react at a detailed level to our purchasing preferences. When I talk about my shopping decisions in my local community, other people are influenced by them, and I am influenced by what my friends and neighbours tell me in return. That kind of conversation expands exponentially when social media is involved and that is one of the topics explored in the next chapter.

Chapter summary

People are different. Individuals, families, organizations, societies and nations each have their own particular characteristics. Some of these differences are significant enough to become separate categories into which people are grouped: gender, race, class etc. Membership of this kind of category has an enormous influence on what we can and cannot have and do. Other differences form the run-of-the-mill of the daily experience each of us has because of our embeddedness in our particular environment. Negotiating things like who will clear away the breakfast dishes, which car will have right-of-way in a narrow street and who will take responsibility for deciding the advice given to a patient shapes our lives.

We can negotiate the field in which we are currently embedded more effectively when we have as much information as possible about its nature. We discover that information through our senses: what we hear, see, feel, taste and smell, and also by talking to other people about their experience of our shared field. In this way, we influence one another towards change.

Activities

6.1 Individual

Write down ten things that you could do to bring about the change you would like to see. This could be change in your family, work environment or neighbourhood, or generally in the world.

6.2 With another person

Think about either a conversation you had or a social media post that you saw that seemed significant to you. What made it significant? Have you done anything differently because of it? Journal for 5 minutes in response to these questions. Then decide if there is a further conversation you would like to have, or a social media post you would like to make in order to continue this conversation.

6.3 With a group

Has anyone else become involved in the conversation, either in person or on-line? If they have, what difference did that make to the conversation? If nobody else did become involved, what does that mean for you?

Personal reflection

Written by Rachel David (FNTP) Nutritional Therapist

As a child my Mum used to grow her own vegetables and bake her own bread. Meals were a mixture of homemade food and 1970's British pack-aged food, seen by our family as a luxury and a novelty! Sadly, when I was thirteen, my Mum became seriously ill with a brain tumour. Her recovery took many years and my Dad struggled to work, take care of two children and run the home. Food became a quick and convenient process, and as a result I quickly forgot the art of preparing and cooking a nutritious home-made meal. Leaving home at a young age, I did not consider the relationship between food and good health.

Following a car accident, I ended up with chronic pain and headaches. I soon became addicted to opioid painkillers. I also started to struggle with Irritable Bowel Syndrome, and constantly felt exhausted. Gradually I began to experience panic attacks, and the struggle of working and caring for a young child whilst in constant pain became overwhelming. Finally, I suffered a nervous breakdown.

During this period my husband joined a slimming club and brought home a recipe book. We began to use some of the healthy recipes, and I noticed a positive change in my IBS symptoms. I began to read nutrition books and articles, and quickly made the connection between what I had been feeding my body, and the condition of my health. Preparing and eating nutritious food became something positive to focus on during my struggles with mental health, and furthermore I knew the nutrients were supporting my recovery.

I decided to qualify as a Nutritional Therapist so I could help others who were struggling with their health. For over seventeen years now I have been free from the symptoms of IBS and have not struggled with my mental health. Due to these personal experiences, it has made me strongly believe in the benefits of living a holistic lifestyle, particularly ensuring you have the right nutrients to support your body and mind.

Food note

The social conversation around food takes place in the media and on social media. We can watch cookery programmes on television and follow celebrity chefs on Instagram. We can post photographs of our food in exactly the same way they post photographs of theirs (although we may not receive as many 'likes' as they do). Just like food itself, participation has to be regulated.

Previously, I found that social media had made me sick. I force-fed myself on a diet of Instagram and Facebook, believing them to be essential provender for modern life and I became allergic. For a long time since I hit my surfeit, I have avoided the steady 'feed' from the various platforms, turning to and trusting the real-life or vital communication that, anyway, fills my world. Writing this book has made me realize that, in order to influence the dialogue, I need to participate in it.

In Chapter 2, I described how I boil up a pan of different kinds of beans each week and use them in the meals I prepare over the next few days. This week I posted photographs of the process on Instagram, under the hashtag #thisweeksbeans. I soaked hard, pale chickpeas overnight on Tuesday and boiled them on Wednesday. On Thursday I photographed the now plump and golden spheres before I made hummus from some of them and ate it for lunch.

Here is the 'backstory' behind that process. Although it is a bit labour intensive, I prefer chickpeas without their skins, so I follow Yotam Ottolenghi's advice and stir a teaspoon of bicarbonate of soda into the pan with previously soaked chickpeas before I add the plentiful cold water in which I will boil them. I pick the fragile little skins out as I decant the cooked chickpeas into the big plastic box in which I will keep them in the fridge. I store them in their cooking water and scoop them out as needed. I have to say that chickpea skins are a bit like Christmas tree needles in that I keep finding more of them. . .

To make hummus, I whizzed up three or four scoops in my ancient food processor with a garlic clove and a slice of ginger about the size of a ten pence piece, salt, lemon juice, pepper and a little cold water because I wanted my hummus to be quite thin this time. Again, I follow Ottolenghi and serve it slightly warm drizzled in a little bit of warm olive oil in which I have browned some aromatics: more ginger and garlic this time. I ate it with loads of lettuce (my organic veg box had been delivered the day before), some slivers of red onion and a couple of slices of sourdough, piling the warm, fragrant conglomeration on top of the bread and thence into my mouth.

References

Burkeman, O. (2015) *Why can't the world's greatest minds solve the mystery of consciousness?* www.theguardian.com (Accessed 1st October 2019).

Cockman, P., Evans, B. and Reynolds, P. (1992) *Client-centred consulting.* The McGraw-Hill Training Series. Ed. Bennet, R(oger). Maidenhead: McGraw-Hill.

De Beauvoir, S. (1997) *The second sex.* London: Vintage.

Eddo-Lodge, R. (2018) *Why I'm no longer talking to white people about race.* London: Bloomsbury.

Gilligan, C. (1982) *In a different voice.* USA: Harvard University Press.

Kaur, O. (2010) Personal communication.

Korn, L. (2016) *Nutrition essentials for mental health.* New York: Norton.

Lawson, N. (2020) *Cook, eat, repeat.* London: Chatto & Windus.

Leyse-Wallace, R. (2008) *Linking nutrition to mental health.* New York: iUniverse.

Littlewood, R. and Lipsedge, M. (1989) *Aliens and Alienists: Ethnic minorities and society.* London: Unwin Hyman.

Mayer, E. (2016) *The mind-gut connection.* New York: Harper Collins.

Nevis, E. (1987) *Organizational consulting.* Cleveland: Gestalt Institute of Cleveland Press.

Orbach, S. (1988) *Fat is a feminist issue.* London: Arrow.

Parlett, M. (1991) 'Reflections on field theory', *British Gestalt Journal*, 1(2), pp. 69–81.
Perls, F., Hefferline, R.F. and Goodman, P. (1992 [1951]) *Gestalt therapy: Excitement and growth in the human personality*. London: Souvenir Press.
Ryde, J. (2009) *Being white in the helping professions*. London: Jessica Kingsley.
Toklas, A.B. (1983) *The Alice B. Toklas cook book*. London: Brilliance Books.
Wheeler, G. (2019) EAGT conference. Budapest.
Wilber, K. (2006) *Integral spirituality*. Boston: Integral Books.

7 Vital and virtual

Personal and digital relationships

Introduction

In this chapter, I am exploring the contrasts between embodied, here-and-now, 'in real-life' experiences that are 'vital' because they are immediate and embodied, and those that are 'virtual' because they are mediated through a screen. The digital world continues to extend ever more fully and seamlessly into our day-to-day experience. Awareness of the way we identify, define and differentiate between direct experience and that mediated by a screen then becomes increasingly important, both for individuals and as a society. Understanding the dynamics of the interface with the digital world for ourselves, as health professionals, allows us to be more effective in noticing its potential impact on the mental health of our clients.

Increasing use of digital methods of communication also means that many of us will be changing the way we contact and interact with our clients. There is an opportunity here to refine how we work and offer a more efficient and effective service. For this reason, part of this chapter is devoted to exploring the on-line experience of accessing essential services. While our day-to-day work takes place in specific, limited contexts like offices, clinics and wards, it has a significant impact on wider society. We have codes of ethics that reflect the values we bring to our work. Some practitioners (including me) consider that 'the job' brings some kind of social responsibility with it, which is why I believe that paying attention to the wider social sphere, which is the context in which we work, is essential.

To begin to underline why this discussion is relevant for health professionals, here is a glimpse of what happened while I was working therapeutically with a young man who was searching for the direction his life would take. We talked about sex. He told me about his sexual experience with partners he had met socially and also about his on-line sexual experiences, which happened much more frequently. From many similar conversations, I know well that it is as common now for some people to express their sexuality in a way that is mediated through a screen as it is to do so in the flesh, so I accepted what he said quite casually. He seemed relieved about this, and we went on to explore the similarities and differences of his experience. He decided that in the flesh was more satisfying, but on-screen was easier and did bring its own satisfactions. I will pick up this theme later.

DOI: 10.4324/9781003172161-8

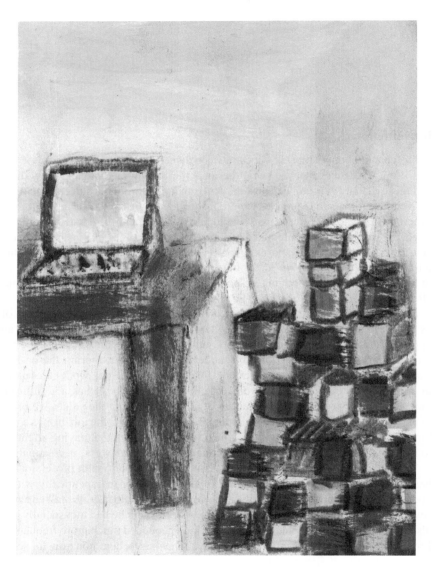

Making it count

A large section of the chapter is devoted to economics and perhaps I need to justify why I think it fits here. Earlier, in Chapter 5, I described how food is being traded digitally using derivatives, essentially financial packages the value of which comes from what someone else would pay for them at the time of selling. This kind of notional, digital trading creates a system in which monetary value becomes disconnected from things that have value in themselves, like a piece of land, or a field of crops or a plate of food. Economics has a direct effect on the mental (and physical) health of the population because it influences the distribution of wealth and, consequently, access to healthy food and other essentials for life. In earlier chapters, I have described the effect on mental health of our current attitudes to food, and how diet is connected to depression, autism, dementia and other diseases that are becoming more common, so the link between economics and health is quite a direct one. Economics also impacts on the use of the natural resources we need to grow heathy food. Modern production and distribution methods are dedicated to producing as much as possible so that it can be sold for profit. This is how 'the market' works. I believe that we need to approach our economic and political choices with a very clear sense of what has real value for human beings now and make that distinct from the hunger just to have more which is intrinsic to current system, despite how devastating the real cost of that approach is to the natural environment and to human wellbeing.

It seems that in the UK, and in other parts of the developed world, we have accepted a food production and distribution system that does not nourish our bodies in the way that we need and can actually harm our health (processed food, refined carbohydrates, trans fats, etc.). At the same time, it is exploiting animals, destroying eco-systems and depleting the soil, consequently threatening the continued existence of our species. Living with these facts, or somehow managing to live in denial of them challenges our mental health as much as it jeopardizes our physical health. Returning to the conversation with my client, it seems possible to draw a comparison between attitudes to sex and food here. Like digital sex, processed food is sufficiently tasty, satisfying enough and, above all, easy to come by. Yet a diet of only 'digital' food does not provide profound satisfaction or deep nourishment. Neither does it bring the next generation into being.

Rather reluctantly, in this chapter I feel like I have to mention the attempts to produce synthetic food that are taking place. These digital 'foodstuffs' fill me with horror, as does the greed and hubris involved in the attempt. Genetic engineering of food plants is also a lively current topic that I believe has a place in this chapter. It is interesting that, in an effort to resolve the world's problems with food, somehow it is easier to think about replacing how we traditionally grow it with a new system, rather than making the current system fit for purpose. It is an issue for society because these initiatives are connected with making a profit for investors and, in my view, anyway, that kind of approach has not served us well so far. Health professionals are likely to be interested in this topic from the point of view of whether it can provide proper nutrition for people and, also whether as a system, it can be trusted. After all, food is a necessity of life for all of us.

Throughout the book, I have been highlighting how our personal and societal relationships with food parallel our relationships with the world in general. Consequently, the appetite we have for data and the way we process it has relevance for the whole picture. The ability to regulate intake effectively is important for a healthy relationship with food (see Chapter 3) and also for managing the overload of input from social media in particular, which is stressful for many people. Stress has been recognized as a contributory factor to anxiety and depression (Korn, 2016). In this chapter I explore the different kinds of nourishment available from information, how we regulate our intake (or not) and what that means for us in the context of our flesh and blood relationships and ongoing life choices.

Artificial Intelligence is increasingly part of our environment: digital assistants like Siri and Alexa are available as constant companions, we interact with chatbots during many of our phone calls and robots are involved in production and distribution of the things we use. Intelligence is part of mental health, so it is important for health professionals to consider what, if anything is the difference between human intelligence and Artificial Intelligence? I offer some ways of thinking about this in the chapter.

Finally, I look at how health professionals use on-line working, its plusses and minuses. Our clients and ourselves have participated in a digital revolution which was intensified in the pandemic by the need to keep a physical distance from one another. So, we had to find an effective way of doing our jobs on-line and needed to do that really quickly. Now the in-real-life world is opening up, we face different choices. We have the opportunity to renegotiate the balance between face-to-face meetings and digital contact that works most effectively for our clients and ourselves which, hopefully, also contributes to the quality of mental health of society as a whole.

Economics for eaters

One of the central tasks of government is to make sure that the people have enough to eat. Whether Marie Antoinette did actually say, 'Let them eat cake' or not, the French Revolution happened, and there were riots connected with food in Britain too in the eighteenth century. At the beginning of the Covid pandemic, when supermarket shelves were empty, all of us had a taste of fear, panic and the compulsion to compete for scarce, but essential resources. The financial crash of 2008 showed us what can happen when market structures fail. The world was barely recovering from that when the pandemic hit us. It is pretty well accepted now that the crossover of the virus from animals to humans took place in a food market, or at least has some association to the dangers associated with increasingly large-scale food distribution practices. We know that something similar (or maybe even worse) will happen if we cannot change how the food and financial markets, which are closely linked, are organized. Many health professionals have been involved in responding to the physical and mental health needs of clients and patients throughout the pandemic and are likely to continue to have to respond for a number of years to come. Thinking about the political and economic aspects that underlie what has happened may help us make sense of it for ourselves and, potentially, influence our own political and economic choices, and the way that we involve ourselves in society. It may also give us some insight that we can apply usefully in our work.

In Chapter 5, I described the growth of the societal structures that have arisen out of our need to eat and I begin this exploration of the connection between food, economics and, subsequently, politics with a brief summary of that section. Over time, the hand-to-mouth existence of hunter-gatherers was gradually replaced by more settled forms of agriculture. With a consistent investment of time, resources and energy into land, the concept of ownership became relevant. What we own affects the quality of life we enjoy. When most of us grew our own food in traditional ways our wealth came from our own skill and hard work as communities of people embedded within our natural environment, akin to the soil, alive to the sources of fresh water and marked by weather. When the direct relationship between day-to-day activity and the acquisition of the nourishment we need to survive was broken, money started to become wealth (Steel, 2020).

The practice of understanding and manipulating money became known as economics. Politics and economics have close links to one another, and the financial policies of political parties follow economic theory. 'Economics is the mother tongue of public policy, the language of public life, and the mindset that shapes society' (Raworth, 2018, p. 6). Most of us need money in order to buy our food and the amount of money we have available to us depends on the political system we have voted for. For me, the link between politics and food, and the consequent impact on the mental and physical health of society, has become really clear, whether those political decisions are about land use in the eighteenth century, pesticide use in the twentieth, or free school meals in the twenty-first century.

The 2008 Financial Crash made me begin to wonder about the economic system we use. The crash was so sudden and unexpected that I, as an ordinary person who had never studied economics, wondered how it could be that all the assumptions and structures on which our financial (and political) systems were founded, and all the theories that had been developed over centuries, could be so shattered by events. I was working with a post-graduate economics student at the time. At our first meeting following the crash we named what had happened and then stared dumbly at one another. I felt that, in his place, I would have a sense of the ground falling out from under me. It seemed to me that all the knowledge he had gained had suddenly become useless and meaningless, and wondered (not out loud) if he experienced any of that disillusionment himself. I explored the situation with him as tactfully as I could. Some of the feelings and reactions he spoke about were similar to those I described, although he said little about how he was being affected and it seemed like his full response was still unfolding. As we spoke together, he looked young and in dismay. But the academic structures are strong, and a lot of money, power and status has been invested in them so, pretty soon, things just started to go on as usual again. My client was not the only person whose mental health was affected by the financial crash. World events impact on us all, and the Covid pandemic is another, more recent reminder of the effect of political and economic choices.

While I had lost faith in capitalism after 2008, there seemed to be no workable alternative. I decided to explore the situation more deeply in order to make some sense of it for myself, but also so that I was in a position to work on it with clients for whom the issue was relevant. Eventually, I found the book 'Postcapitalism' (2015) by Paul Mason. He revisited some of the ideas of Karl Marx and they seemed plausible. But I had lived through the era of the Soviet Union and I had seen how making everyone workers in the systems of production, together with powerful state intervention, created different inequalities and new hierarchies for the people. The eventual disintegration of the Soviet Union seemed to prove to everyone that this kind of communism does not work. Back then in the 1980s, the world was left with only one superpower, the USA, and this was when capitalism and neo-liberalism began to prevail in the west.

Towards the end of the second decade of the twenty-first century, as I began to explore fresh approaches to politics and economics, I could see the fault lines in the current system. The traditional approaches seemed to be no longer relevant in the context of climate change, and in a world in which a growing majority of people had access to a smartphone. From around that time, I was able to see and talk to my friends in Italy over Skype whenever I liked, and at no cost. Mass gatherings of people were able to be organized with a few hours' notice through Facebook. Activists and terrorists, as well as ordinary people, could be in constant touch with one another via the devices in their homes, bags and pockets. Responding to changes as fundamental as these had an effect on the mental health of individuals and communities. I knew this because I had seen it in my consulting room, as well as experiencing it myself.

I became dubious about large, centralized, bureaucratic, authoritative, repressive regimes in which the system itself becomes more important than the people. I saw traces of those characteristics in many political systems in the world whether they inhabited the left, the right or the middle ground. In the west, the pursuit of constant financial growth is costly for social cohesion and planetary resources. As individuals, and as a society, we face difficult choices. Can we change enough to avoid further environmental exploitation and re-direct wealth from the affluent who have more money than they can ever need to those who are hungry? Can we even change enough to avoid another pandemic, being that food-related practices are seen by science as being a contributory cause?

Anxiety about the future, and particularly about access to work, food and adequate housing is likely to remain a long-term mental health issue for many people. This kind of mental health issue cannot be addressed by the individual, but only by taking action as communities, and as a society. Thinking about the issues and gaining some knowledge about potential ways of addressing them, enables health professionals to work with clients in a more resourced way around these concerns.

While I have not yet seen any developments in political systems that might offer a potentially viable way of moving the world away from the brink of catastrophe, I have discovered a new approach to economics that seems hopeful. I believe it is relevant for health professionals to be informed about innovative alternative approaches because, while each of us has our own political views, this kind of knowledge provides more flexibility to respond to matters that concern our clients, and to the wider society in which we all participate.

Doughnut economics

In her (2018) book, economist Kate Raworth offers both a rationale for why old economic models have become obsolete and a compellingly argued new model of a system to replace them. The 'Doughnut' is the image she uses to bring all her ideas together, she sometimes also refers to it as a compass. The diagram she uses resembles a ring doughnut with, nestled inside it where the doughnut's hole would be, the basic needs for humanity which range from water and food to justice and equality, form the spokes of an invisible inner wheel. On the outside of the ring the basic needs for the planet radiate out: fresh air, pure water, healthy soil and species diversity (which are all what humans need to survive too). The Doughnut itself is the 'sweet-spot' (2018, p. 45) where the needs of both planet and people can be recognized and met. It is 'both an ecologically safe and socially just space for humanity' (p. 45).

In order to achieve this goal, Raworth proposes replacing the striving for continual growth which is the aim of capitalism with finding a balance between meeting the essential needs of the people and avoiding the unsustainable exploitation of the planet. In this scenario, the pre-eminence of 'the market' could be replaced by what she calls an 'Embedded Economy' (p. 71) in which needs are the driving force rather than profit. She describes how the activities of the market (the exchange of food and other essentials for life between those who produce them and those who need them) can become embedded in a system in which government, business, trade and finance can make a contribution towards achieving the goals of fairness and sustainability. In this system meeting needs, those of the people and those of the environment, would replace making profit.

This kind of economy also takes into account the contribution each household makes to the wider society, which is a welcome recognition. Raworth calls the household the core economy. She recounts that the unmarried Adam Smith, author of 'The Wealth of Nations', one of the core texts in the evolution of economics moved back home to live with his mother Margaret Douglas when he began writing it (p. 79). He failed to notice how her effort and productivity was essential for enabling his, and so did not acknowledge it in his book. The unpaid care provided in the household is still a blind spot for economic theory.

Imagine a society in which a household was a contributor rather than a consumer. Of course, households already contribute to society by nurturing citizens and enabling them to work and participate in society and the economy. Making sure children turn up at school to be educated and that workers are clothed, fed and ready to carry out the requirements of their money-earning activity, whatever that may be, are household responsibilities.

Working from home has become more widespread because of the pandemic and the trend is likely to continue. Raworth talks about the desktops and laptops, smartphones and tablets, and the digital connections needed to use them as 'distributed capital'. She observes that 'Anyone with an internet connection can entertain, inform, learn and teach worldwide. Every household, school or business rooftop can generate renewable energy' (p. 192). Homes could become centres of livelihood again, just as they were in pre-industrial times and as Raworth says, 'blur the divide between producers and consumers, allowing everyone to become a prosumer, both a maker and a user in the peer-to-peer economy' (p. 192). These ideas reflect the renegotiation between home and work that is already under way and affirm it as a viable alternative. Bringing possible solutions closer to home empowers individuals to take action. A sense of agency in dealing with challenges really helps with maintaining mental health.

Raworth also acknowledges the importance of 'the commons', the natural or digital spaces which all can access and also make contributions towards, and that are self-organizing. In nature it might reflect the system of common land that provided sustenance for communities centuries ago, and still does to an extent even today. In the digital realm we call them the 'creative commons' and they include the platforms Wikipedia and YouTube as well as more specialist sources, all of which organize themselves in response to the use that is made of them. Raworth refers to the Nobel Prize winning work of political scientist Elinor Ostrom (1999) which involved identifying natural commons that worked well and finding out what it was that made them successful. She found that they 'were governed by clearly defined communities with collectively agreed rules and punitive sanctions for those who broke them' (Raworth, 2018, p. 83). In these circumstances, natural commons 'can turn out to be a triumph, outperforming both state and market in sustainably stewarding and equitably harvesting Earth's resources'.

Maybe we need to create more commons, and also recognize more of those that are already in place. Community run initiatives that are available in my area include a 'Repair Cafe' where people can bring broken items and a 'Library of Things' which lends infrequently used items like tools and small appliances when they are needed. Both schemes offer a platform for the resources of the community to be shared, whether they are objects or know-how. They are run by volunteers so locals can experience the results of their participation, and also choose how much and how to be involved. Contributing to the wellbeing of our community is seen as rewarding in itself, which has an effect on the mental health of participants. Schemes organize themselves in response to the resources of commitment, time and expertise invested in them, so are flexible and responsive by nature. If one activity becomes unnecessary or uninteresting it will naturally decline and be replaced by something new. These kinds of community-run projects are found in many areas. Much of the societal response to Covid came from neighbourhood self-help groups, often centred around the provision of food, who mobilized quickly in the first lockdown and made a significant contribution to community morale.

This dynamic is in tune with Field Theory, which was introduced in the previous chapter. As discussed there, fields have their own ways of continually unfolding, and reorganizing in response to subtle shifts within them. In the examples of successful natural commons she researched, Ostrom (2012 in Raworth, 2018) identified the need for mutually agreed rules to be in place in order for the organization to regulate itself. These may be informally agreed, often unspoken, guidelines that emerge from actually doing the activity (Field Theory) or formally agreed written procedures, or anything in between. The important thing for me seems to be that the system has the ability to address conflict in a healthy and creative way and I return to this point in the final chapter.

Raworth advocates an approach to economics that is less mechanical and more agricultural, preferring metaphors of complex, diverse organisms rather than those of cause-and effect-mechanisms. In her ideal economic scenario, the classical approach to pollution – that the technology to sort it out will eventually develop – is replaced by an attitude of avoiding pollution and other environmental harm, in accordance with the principles of the 'Doughnut'.

Other approaches that offer an alternative to the way economics operates in the west will, no doubt, continue to become available. I like this one because it focuses on areas that seem to me to be important for change and is in tune with the change models that are connected with the theoretical underpinnings of my profession. They reflect what I already see emerging around me too. I also like it because it is organized around a metaphor that is related to food. Maybe a different model would fit better for you, but knowing what alternatives exist may offer a fresh perspective on the society in which we and our clients live. This can help us to serve them better and also provide an opportunity to contribute towards creating more options for everyone.

Case study – the ethical independent grocer

Written by Jo Shah, Independent Grocer, Penarth.

I opened my Organic food shop after 5 months of travelling around Europe with my husband Neill. On our travels we had been dining off locally grown fresh produce. As we were both interested in the impact of food production on the environment, we were keen to minimize food miles wherever possible. We are in South Wales and as much as possible we buy from Wales. Where we do buy imported goods, we make sure that nothing is air freighted and that they travel to us by sea. Two of our wholesalers are Cooperatives with strong ethical beliefs in line with our own. Unfortunately, to survive as a small producer, wholesalers are the only way of getting the products to market. This has proved frustrating on a number of occasions when products are travelling from West Wales and bypassing our town to be re distributed from a wholesaler back to us. One specific example of this is a butter produced in West Wales, bought by a wholesaler in Bristol and then driven back to Cardiff. If we had bought the same butter from our other supplier, it would have travelled up to Yorkshire and then back to us! For this reason, I have stopped buying this product and chosen a butter made more locally to Bristol as it makes more road mile sense. With fresh, locally grown vegetables this isn't a problem, but the same issue has arisen with meat. Our Welsh, organic meat supplier is in Mid Wales yet some of the meat they distribute comes from the next town to us. With the growth of farmers markets some of these issues can be addressed but I think in what is an extremely competitive market, effective food distribution is an issue.

Data hunger

In the last century, an acronym that was used in relation to data processing was GIGO – garbage in, garbage out. I don't hear it these days, but maybe I'm not so much part of those circles now. It seems that this saying is as accurate for humans as it is for computers. As far as our bodies and brains are concerned, eating a healthy diet helps keep us fit and active. For our minds, adequate nourishment and effective regulation of intake are equally necessary for our health, both physical and mental. Here are some ways of thinking about our information diets:

- **Data** the material that surrounds us constantly from our social media, email providers, subscription services (Amazon Prime, Netflix etc), newspapers, television, word-of-mouth.
- **Information** data that might be useful for us currently – that a text message has arrived from a family member, for example.
- **Knowledge** Information we can gather, analyse and use in decision making and communication.
- **Intelligence** Knowing how to acquire and apply knowledge in a way that increases our personal effectiveness and contribution to others, and the ability to do this consistently.
- **Wisdom** Ability to distil profound, universal meaning from experience.

To begin processing, we 'taste' a piece of data, decide whether the flavour seems authentic and nourishing. We 'spit out' anything that seems to us like 'fake news', lies or propaganda, whatever we consider those things to be. Just like the choco-late fudge cake that seems so appetizing to sight and smell, with some data that is available to us we may think we want it, but it is not so wholesome for us once we've swallowed it, and it sits heavily and acidly in our stomach for hours after-wards. After this initial processing, data that is proved to be useful and nourish-ing becomes information. We ingest a mixed diet of information which produces knowledge (energy would be the food equivalent) and the nutrients we need to maintain ourselves and grow in intelligence (proteins, fats, vitamins etc.). This whole process is the diet that provides the potential to be wise.

So far, I have been focusing on the way an individual processes available mate-rial but, of course, we have processes for potentially converting data to wisdom as a society too. Academic literature is a good example here. Every step and con-tribution to the body of knowledge associated with each discipline is critically reviewed and checked, so that its authenticity (nutritional value) is established. The libraries and databases that are the vital and virtual products of the system exist as the ground of future learning. They are the foundation for the ingenuity that is needed to enable the brilliant leaps of perception that underlie significant scientific advances. The speed with which vaccines against Covid-19 were pro-duced is a powerful recent example of how a skilfully constructed body of knowl-edge can be used.

Newspapers, both on-line and on paper, and broadcast news bulletins are cor-roborated accounts of events, plus analysis and comment. 'Newspaper of Record' is a term that previously used to be heard more than it is now. It is used to describe an authoritative, trusted, transparent provider of information.

Shared sources of information are part of the shared culture of a society. In current times, we have the ongoing sharing of information that is social media. Field Theory (Chapter 6) tells us that knowing more about the nature and dynamics of the of the forces that connect us help us to negotiate them more effectively. That being the case, it is probably important to assess the material that comes to us in this way to decide if it is relevant, useful sustenance or an excess of empty calories, and to support our clients to do likewise, where that is appropriate.

Virtual food

Cellular meat

The problem is that modern farming practices are cruel to animals, involve clearing rain forests to feed them, thereby harming the environment, and have a harmful effect on the supply of fresh water in the process (Steel, 2020). The answer that some entrepreneurs (including Bill Gates) are proposing is to grow meat in a laboratory. The BBC Food Programme investigated the situation in April 2021 (see Resources section for details) and here is a summary of their findings. The process involves taking a cell from a living or dead animal (chickens, pigs, insects. . .) and, in a vessel called a bioreactor, feeding that cell with the nutrients it needs to divide many millions of times and eventually, to resemble a piece of meat. A potential benefit of this method of production, if it can be done at a small enough scale, is that the product can be grown in facilities close to where large numbers of people need food, like refugee camps and deprived urban areas. A possible undesirable consequence might be that the energy and land use required to produce food for the cell might be the same, or greater than that needed to feed an actual chicken or pig. . .

Genome editing

Once again, for the current situation at the time of writing, I'm referring to the BBC Food Programme (details in the Resources section). Genome editing can be used in plants and animals. It is different from the Genetic Modification approach that was so controversial a few years ago. It is more specific and selective, and the effects of the process can be bred out within a generation. E.U. rules had prohibited its use but, since Brexit, the English Government has been keen to adopt it and so a public consultation has taken place which closed in March 2021. The argument they make is that the process is equivalent to the natural selective breeding techniques that have been commonly used. I am specifying the English government here because food is a devolved matter, so the governments here in Wales, and in Scotland and Northern Ireland will make their own decisions. A potential benefit of the method is that it is possible to develop new species that could be more easily grown near cities.

A drawback of both these approaches is that the desire to make money is a driving factor. The drive to make a profit has not so far resulted in a food production and distribution system that encourages a healthy diet and lifestyle, or a healthy planet. I am concerned that 'when you do what you've always done, you always get what you always got'.

Artificial Intelligence and human intelligence

I can scarcely believe that I am about to discuss my experience of conversations with Siri and Alexa, two concepts that exist only in the noughts and ones of the microprocessors of my smartphone. Yet I know that it is certainly possible to talk something into being, in fact conversation is one of the commonest ways of bringing anything about. This book began with experiences: a sip of rosato wine (it came into existence in the winemaker's head, she told me), a mouthful of cheese in a high village, a story about a walnut and a chickpea. . . . The sensations and emotions associated with these experiences became food for thought and then an idea emerged. At that point, the conversations became more intense. Is it interesting, worthwhile? Does it offer a fresh perspective? Will anyone want it? A book is as much an invention of telling and listening as it is pages inscribed with symbols that have been bound together.

We are already accustomed to accessing virtual realms that are not digital at all. This makes us fertile ground for digital simulations. I ask Siri to time 20 minutes for me and he (my instinct is to ascribe gender to 'voice') responds cheerfully and obligingly. I feel the light, momentary satisfaction that comes with a successful transaction and settle into my meditation. No satisfaction for Siri, however, and no frustration either, although I often get frustrated by the seeming 'stupidity' of digital assistants. Humans are relational beings. We survive in relationship with our environment, so our reaction to satisfying or annoying exchanges with elements of it has significance for us. We know we are alive from these interactions, and we learn from them how to handle similar experiences in the future. I have learned to say 'Alexa' very loudly and clearly, and then wait for a response before I say, 'Play Argentine Tango'. If anything goes wrong, I have to adjust my approach because the system is unable to do adjust its. Yet. Technology moves very quickly, so it may not be long before digital assistants actually become useful. Someone makes the machines, and it is important that we pay attention to whom the image and likeness in which they are made belongs. There is a danger of defaulting to male, white and western assumptions again here. This has significance because we (humans) will adapt along with the machines, since that is what we do. That may lead to a very interesting future but like with any interaction, digital ones are probably best approached with awareness of where they are leading us. Health professionals work with human beings. Awareness of how interacting with digital simulations influences our human encounters may offer some useful insights for our work with clients.

'Stroke' theory

I mentioned Transactional Analysis, founded by Eric Berne, in Chapter 4. Here is another theory associated with it. In this context, a 'stroke' is an acknowledgement of one person by another, or others. Human beings need this recognition to survive, literally when we are vulnerable – I'm thinking of patients in Intensive Care Units (I've been doing that a lot over previous months) and children, of course – and we all need it emotionally too. We need recognition so much that, if we fail to receive positive 'strokes', like a warm verbal response, a greeting or a smile, we will go all out for any reaction we can, even if it is a negative one like a refusal, or a scowl, or being told to sit on the naughty step. . . . There are 'strokes' for doing, 'That meal was delicious'. And strokes for just being like having our eyes met by someone we love, being told someone is proud of us, or having cold hands rubbed by warm ones. . . . Human beings thrive in response to this kind of recognition, Artificial Intelligence is oblivious to it.

Robots

The potential is there for machines to do the tasks humans don't like, or don't want to do. Some of the activities we may not like to do include the things we get paid for. We earn the money to buy the food and shelter we need, and to provide ourselves with the means for enjoyment, from activities that, in themselves, might sometimes seem boring, mundane and meaningless. All jobs have some uncongenial aspects yet, because we have to have to do them (and this is what humans are like) we make some kind of meaning from it. Depending on the sorts of jobs we do, different satisfactions are available to us. We enjoy the camaraderie that comes from working with others; the kindness and the humour and, above all, the sense of belonging. We enjoy the financial rewards; working hard for long hours and watching the bank account grow. We enjoy the sense of making a difference to others, to service, devotion and the satisfaction of perceiving the outcomes of our actions. We like power and status. In his book, 'Kitchen Confidential' (2010), New York chef Anthony Bourdain described with pride the swashbuckling tenacity with which chefs in busy restaurant kitchens approached their work. The long hours, burning heat, hard physical work and expectations of demanding customers were accepted as a rite of passage into an elite brotherhood.

Our sense of who we are is deeply connected with the work we do. What happens if someone else decides that our job would be better done by a robot? In my job, I feel insulated from that because the whole point of it is to explore what it means to be human with another person. Yet many on-line questionnaires and programmes exist that people use successfully for addressing issues that are troubling them, including depression and anxiety. I found this self-help guide easily when I searched the internet:

www.nhsinform.scot/illnesses-and-conditions/mental-health/mental-health-self-help-guides/depression-self-help-guide.

Medical professionals are being aided in diagnosis by Artificial Intelligence. See:

www.nhsx.nhs.uk/ai-lab/ for more information.

Already on-line equivalents for face-to-face meetings are commonplace. The pandemic has forced us in this direction. The equivalents may be a phone consultation or a Zoom session in real time, or they may be accessed through websites at the user's convenience. Pressures on the health service make it likely this trend will continue and develop further even when meeting in person becomes safer. Our clients will be facing the impact of these kind of changes to the world of work in their lives too. Thinking about the implications of this may further resource us for our work with them.

I saw for myself how a robot can be used while on a visit to the marble cutting factory that belongs to my friend, Arianna Marchetti. Her business is in Carrara, in north west Italy. Carrara has been a centre for quarrying and working marble from ancient times, and its product has been used for many landmark buildings all over the world, including the Pantheon and Marble Arch. The day I visited it the hangar-like space was peaceful but full of intent. The great cutting machines stood ready and finished goods were boxed up and marked with the Marchetti logo awaiting transport to wherever in the world they were going. The most consistent movement in the whole space was the robot. Silent and relentless, it carried out its tasks, oblivious to observers and mindless of time.

How different this was from the sculpture studios in the centre of town. I had read about the famous Nicoli studios in 'Honey from a Weed' by Patience Grey. Her biographer Adam Federman describes her as a 'Visionary Food Writer' in the sub-title of his (2017) book 'Fasting and Feasting' Her partner was a sculptor, and they spent some time in Carrara together in 1962.

> You have to imagine this 19th century piazza, the buildings of stone with the stucco parts painted in chrome and bulls' blood. These colours when first applied stood up to the dazzling white of the mountains in the background; now faded, to tones of pink and gold. A stout Victorian palace rose up at the western end, looking at the marble mountains. Adjoining it at right-angles loomed a studio of immense size built for the execution of colossal marbles.
>
> (Grey, 2009, p. 39)

Now, colossal marbles are produced by machines programmed with instructions for cutting putti (disembodied angels) or acanthus leaves, rather than hot, dusty humans with chisels and hammers – and with thirsts which are slaked, in camaraderie, at the bar over the road. . .

Whether we regret the loss of some of the work done originally 'by hand' or rejoice in it, there are implications: 'the significance of this revolution for work, wages and health hinges on how digital technologies are owned and used' (Raworth, 2018, p. 191). If robots make the things that make the money, there is potential for far greater inequality between people than there is already. The owners of the capital that finances the robots will make a profit and the workers will be out of a job. How to avoid this catastrophe? 'Doughnut' Economist Kate Raworth suggests changes to the tax system: 'Switch from taxing labour to taxing the use of non-renewable resources' (p. 193) and 'At the same time, invest more in skilling people up where they beat robots hands-down: in creativity, empathy, insight and human contact'. These attributes are what we as health professionals use in our work. They are also how families and communities provide environments that support mental health for us all.

Professionals on-line

Even before the Covid pandemic forced many of us into staying at home, remote working was becoming recognized as a trend. I have been observing, and reflecting on, how accessing work (and other activities) supported by digital technology at home has suddenly become part of our lives. In doing so, it has become clear to me that things will not go back to being the same as they were before. Consequently, we will probably all need to discover how to do our own work most effectively using a blend of on-line and in-person approaches. Some readers may also be working within organizations that are in the process of figuring out how best to manage the balance between face-to-face and on-line working, and they might be expected to make a contribution to how it evolves there. This may not seem directly connected with the topic of food and mental health, but it is certainly relevant for how practitioners in the field may approach undertaking their work.

Sketching in some of the background to the rise of digital working may be helpful for approaching how the situation develops in an informed way. In their review of what they call 'teleworking', Lamond, Daniels and Standen (2005) revisit previous work on the characteristics of jobs that were commonly being done remotely at that time (Daniels, Lamond and Standen, 2001). They identify certain features that are important for understanding the nature of the work being undertaken and how it can be done effectively:

- Knowledge. How much the worker needs to know in order to carry out the role effectively
- Technology requirement. Computers, phones, access to systems, internet connection and physical space
- Sphere of contact, understanding the balance between interaction that is mostly within the organization (managers, colleagues) and interaction that is mostly outside it (customers, clients, patients)

Here are some examples from my own recent experience of accessing essential services digitally. Most of them are directly related to a health environment, but I begin with a description of contacting the tax office. I think describing the contrast between them helps to provide a clearer perspective.

The tax officer

I called HMRC (the people who calculate and collect income tax from me directly because I am self-employed) to query a demand for a payment. The call was picked up by an automated system that asked me the reason for my call and for some identification information. The system told there were delays because of difficulties caused by the pandemic which meant a response might take longer than usual, and I was put on hold. The helpful man I spoke to after not too long a wait was working from home. I know this because we could both hear children in the background at one point, and so he explained why. He clearly had fast access to my digital tax records and was consequently absolutely certain that I did have to pay the amount requested, explaining the reasons for it and making an effort to be sure I understood. Unfortunately, I was convinced so had to pay up, which I did by means of an electronic transfer directly from my bank account.

The GP surgery

I thought it was past the time that I should have been called for my Covid vaccination and rang my GP surgery to check what was happening. After quite a few minutes of listening to a voice telling me I was second in the queue, I reached the top of the pile but had to wait still longer before my GP's recorded voice explained that I needed to ring back after 2pm if I was expecting test results or, alternatively, write a letter, or access the website if I wanted a repeat prescription. If I continued to hold (and my call was very important to them), I would be responded to by a staff member to whom I should explain the reason for my call. She said there were other health professionals like nurses, dieticians and physiotherapists who worked alongside the GP and who may be the appropriate source of treatment for me, and that the receptionist would help me to be directed to the appropriate person. In the event, when I did eventually get through, the receptionist herself was able to check my records. She told me that they still held details of an old address and telephone number, which meant they had not been able to contact me. I was told to write a letter, giving my old and new addresses and drop it into the surgery, which I did. It then took another call, and another journey through the answering procedure, to get my updated information and myself on to the list for the injection, although I received the jab only a few days later.

The orthopaedic surgeon

I was due for a 3-yearly check-up following an operation and received a letter to say it would take place over the telephone. I agreed to this and was given a specific date and time for the call. The surgeon rang me himself. He listened to my experiences and concerns and suggested I came in for an x-ray at a later date. I was invited by letter to attend at the hospital several weeks later, at which point I met my surgeon at social distance and with both of us wearing masks, to discuss my post-operative state.

Analysis – a service user's subjective experience

The tax officer was working at home, with access to, I guess, the digital self-assessment tax records of everyone in the country and also having the knowledge and expertise to interpret the information he accessed and explain it to someone with limited technical knowledge, but with quite an emotional investment in the outcome.

The receptionist was working in the surgery building. I suppose the telephone answering and information service was meant to help her deal with a high level of incoming calls by filtering out some of them in accordance with the surgery's administrative preferences. She was able to access at least the contact details part of my medical records. I cannot tell whether she also had access to details of the issues that had brought me to visit my GP over the years. I notice that I would very much prefer that she did not have access to those records. Although there is nothing scandalous there and, in fact, not much there at all, she does not have the knowledge to understand the information, or any expertise that might be of help to me in resolving my symptoms. Probably more importantly, she is not bound by any codes of ethics around how to use the information (if she does have access to it). When I visit the surgery, I meet her face-to-face, and she lives in the neighbourhood and is likely to know people who know me, so I have to rely on her judgement and discretion.

The secretary of the surgeon has access to my contact details and also to some case details that have appeared in letters sent to me previously. I do not know if she has access to full case details and x-rays. The surgeon himself has intimate knowledge, having cut open my body while I was unconscious. Knowledge, then can be further categorized:

Types of knowledge

- **Factual information**. Details that may be more or less personal to the client (patient, caller, service user, taxpayer, customer, etc.). Health professionals are likely to have access to more personal information than, say, internet service providers who only know an address and the type of modem or router used, although they do have access to bank account details too.
- **Professional expertise**. Training and experience that is relevant to the client's need: how to interpret a tax statement; how to update an address record and how to arrange for an injection to be administered (although possibly not able to achieve both tasks in one stage); how to perform an operation and tell if it is 'successful' within accepted professional parameters. Health professionals are likely to have high levels of professional expertise although we may often be supported by people who do not.
- **Ability to relate to and communicate effectively with others**. I was convinced I needed to pay the tax and did so; I arrived at the appropriate place and time to meet the nurse who was there ready with a syringe and so I acquired some protection from Covid; I know that the surgeon is satisfied with the results of the operation.

The various outcomes of my activities were achieved satisfactorily. I notice I still have feelings about all these interactions, which may possibly be discerned by sensitive readers. This is significant because it seems natural that, as humans, we bring our pre-conceived ideas into the next situation that seems similar. Our perceptions and reactions in the new encounter will be coloured by our previous experience and this may affect both the tone and the outcome.

Vital and virtual – effective interactions

All these kinds of knowledge are needed for face-to-face interactions as well as digital ones. Information is often accessed digitally in real-life situations too now, so it can be present via a computer terminal on a desk. Nevertheless, the ability to relate to and communicate with the client or user is likely to be different in vital and virtual situations. The tax officer could not point to areas of the calculations to help me understand how they worked and had to gauge how much I was understanding of what he was saying by my verbal cues, tone of voice, rhythm of responding etc. because he could not see my face. The surgeon also had to pick up verbal clues from me during our telephone call, although we were both able to see the x-rays on the computer screen and tune into each other's facial and body reactions during our face-to-face meeting. I feel like the aim for the receptionist was just to process my call as soon as possible and move on the next patient. As a result, our communication was very transactional, and I had to stop her a few times from ending the call before my questions had been fully answered. This might be considered appropriate, because her role was mainly to route enquiries elsewhere, within a system that was too complex for the process to be fully automated. In this respect, she worked very closely in tune with the technology.

In order to focus more fully on the technology aspect of digital communication and, particularly, home working, I would like to introduce a different case study.

The admin. section

Working in an academic healthcare context, this group of around half a dozen women takes care of administrative functions, scheduling appointments and resolving day-to-day hitches to organizational systems, both computerized and clerical. Their 'clients' are the managers of the organization, academics and students. They usually work on-site, in a busy office where colleagues can 'pop-in' to discuss any issues personally and informally. When the pandemic required all of them to work from home, things changed.

Some of the team liked working at home, others did not. The factors that were relevant to their responses included personal circumstances, whether they lived alone or with others who might support or make demands on them (home-schooling children, for example). Their natural personal style also had an effect – the 'introverts' liked being insulated to some extent from the interactions, whereas the more sociable missed the lively atmosphere. The technology the team used in their individual homes was supported by the organization's IT department, who helped with solving the problems they encountered.

Team members communicated one-to-one and in groups with each other and with colleagues from the wider organization to share information and undertake joint problem-solving. There was a strong ethos of support in the team and each member had regular one-to-ones with the line manager, and also team check-ins. Members communicated with each other separately from this, offering mutual friendship and support. A highly-structured return to work programme involving 'bubbles' was put in place when it was permitted.

In this scenario, team-members continued to carry out their activities, only from their own homes. Communication with their 'clients' took place on-line rather than in person and there was flexibility around who could communicate with whom and how. Appropriate technology support was available. A great deal of attention was paid to the personal, emotional experiences of team members and the culture of support that was available in the office moved to on-line. Morale and cohesion remained high throughout.

In the 'Personal Reflection' section towards the end of the chapter, I describe my own experience of the difference between working on-line and meeting face-to-face. When lockdown arrived so suddenly and in such an all-encompassing manner I had to just respond, as did very many other people whose role involved meeting clients regularly in person. Then, afterwards, I reflected on what had happened and arrived at some new insights. In a fast-changing world, this may be the best any of us can do in support of our professional learning.

Having been through a global emergency, there is little appetite now for returning to exactly how things were before, even if it were possible to make that happen. We figure things out as best we can, take what seems like the most appropriate (or sometimes least worst) action, notice what happens and then re-calibrate. This is Field Theory (from Chapter 6) in action. Bringing awareness to the thousands of tiny decisions, adjustments and compromises that form our experience helps us know more about the dynamics of the field we inhabit, allowing us to shape it where we can. For this reason, the 'Activities' section offers a structure and an invitation to do just that. In a fast-moving, complex situation, these kinds of reflective practices keep us up to date with new learning we have gained which, in turn, enables us to work with clients more resourcefully.

Chapter summary

Our food production and supply are deeply embedded in economic and political structures both nationally and internationally. It makes a difference if we think about food as a profitable commodity, or whether we think of it as an essential good that brings benefit to us all: whether it is virtual or vital. Many common mental health issues like stress, anxiety and depression are linked to environmental conditions, particularly access to money. The amount that is available for people to be able buy food and other necessities has a direct relationship with the political and therefore economic choices all of us make in a democratic society. Prioritizing meeting the needs of people, and avoiding exploitation of the environment, rather than aiming for constant economic growth may offer a sustainable way forward.

Casting a thoughtful vote is one way for change to occur. Contributing to the 'conversation' society has about how to move forward is potentially significant too, and social media is an accessible method of reaching into practically every part of our lives: political, social, cultural and culinary. As we participate, it is probably important to differentiate between the types of material to which we are exposed and be discerning about what we choose to integrate. This kind of digital regulation is as important for the mind as food regulation is for the body.

Health professionals are currently negotiating fundamental changes to the balance between face-to-face and on-line contact with our clients, patients, service users, etc. Bringing awareness to the choices we make gives us the opportunity to evaluate the direction in which things are going and adjust them as necessary.

Activities

7.1 Individual

Journal for 10 minutes around how digital communication differs from real-life communication in your experience.

7.2 With one other person

Talk with a colleague (or even with a client if that is appropriate for your profession) either on-line or in person, about the experience in the moment for both of you. Notice if doing this seems to make a difference to the interaction. Maybe even bring what you notice into the discussions.

7.3 Wider context

Your professional association or an organization with whom you work will probably have issued guidelines about on-line working. Re-visit them and decide what you think about them now. Maybe even contribute to some kind of discussion or other opportunity to share learning.

Personal reflection

If you had asked me before the pandemic whether I thought on-line psychotherapy is a good idea, I would have responded with horror. Yet I adapted to it immediately. I suppose that was the consequence of having no choice but to do it if I wanted to continue meeting my clients, and I did. Most of them also wanted to continue meeting me, although a couple of people fell away. We worked out relatively easily between us what kind of platform we would use and, there we were, doing psychotherapy on Skype, or FaceTime or Zoom . . .

We talked about how it was for each of us to be doing it this way. I noticed myself being more personally disclosing than I would be if sitting face-to-face in my own practice room. When I talked about it with my supervisor we wondered if that was some kind of effort to become more present, and I continued to notice the impulse, sometimes discussing with clients how it was for them.

My 'premises' became the background people could see behind my face on the screen. I caught glimpses of people's homes that I never would have had before. It was common for some people to be sitting up on their beds hold-ing a smartphone in front of them when we met. Connection was generally ok, although I always had a 'Plan B' agreed beforehand, often involving a phone call, so without video.

I went on for a while working digitally with people that I had previously met in the flesh. Then someone new asked to work with me, and I had to re-think how I would manage contractual arrangements and agreements that I would normally negotiate through the medium of paper. That was not insurmountable, and I may continue with some aspects of it even when I meet people in the flesh again.

The time for that is approaching and I'm thinking about it. I speak about it with my supervisor almost every time we meet, and we agree that it is important to take things slowly still. I will probably never go back to meeting her face-to-face because the trip to London, which was where we used to meet, took a lot of time, money and effort. So much easier, and equally valuable just to turn on the screen . . .

From this experience I have learned to question absolutes, never say 'never'. By the time they come to me for a substantial 'talking therapy' experience, clients may have looked on the internet and tried some of the many useful self-directed questionnaires or schemes to be found there. I think this may be the future for supporting people with their mental health generally. Material people can access in their own time, and at no cost, could make a big contribution. Talking with another person regularly for fairly substantial amounts of time is likely to become even more 'high-end' than it is already.

Food note

Shopping is like voting. Large corporations pay at least as much attention to the buying habits of consumers as politicians do to the expectations of their constitu-ents. I hear bosses of huge multi-national companies talking on the radio. When they are asked by the interviewer why they are changing their policies to become more environmentally friendly there is a simple answer. It is good for business. While reliance on 'the market' to regulate supply and demand, cost and value has its drawbacks, one benefit is that the everyday choices each of us makes has a direct influence on how companies work.

After a long time watching some people go around the Farmer's Market with shopping baskets and envying how practical they are for keeping cakes or cartons of olives upright, I finally found one I liked in the open-air plant sale I went to on Sunday. Actually, I loved it: handmade from willow, elliptical and with asymmet-ric sides, it seemed like the perfect vessel for an ethical shopper. You can probably see the dilemma coming here. . . . I thought about it carefully. Do I really need more stuff? On balance, I thought that it would make my life (or at least my food-shopping) easier. Also, it seemed to me to symbolize an attitude towards food and commerce with which I wanted to be associated. It was made from environ-mentally friendly, natural materials by an independent, local craftswoman. I was happy to let my money circulate around, bringing benefit to the local economy. So, I joyfully let myself buy it!

References

Bourdain, A. (2010) *Kitchen confidential*. London: Bloomsbury.

Daniels, K., Lamond, D. and Standen, P. (2001) 'Teleworking frameworks for organisational research', *Journal of Management Studies,* 38, pp. 1151–1186.

Federman, A. (2017) *Fasting and feasting: The life of visionary food writer patience grey*. Vermont: Chelsea Green.

Grey, P. (2009) *Honey from a weed*. London: Prospect Books.

Korn, L. (2016) *Nutrition essentials for mental health*. New York: Norton.

Lamond, D., Daniels, K. and Standers, P. (2005) 'Managing virtual workers and virtual organisations', in Holman, D., Wall, T.D., Clegg, Sparrow, P. and Howard, A. (eds.) *The essentials of the new workplace*. Chichester: Wiley.

Mason, P. (2015) *Postcapitalism*. UK: Penguin Random House.

Ostrom, E. (1999) 'Coping with the tragedies of the commons', *Annual Review of Political Science*, 2, pp. 493–535.

Ostrom, E. (2012) Green from the grassroots. *Project Syndicate*, 12 June.

Raworth, K. (2018) *Doughnut economics*. London: Random House Business.

Steel, C. (2020) *Sitopia*. London: Chatto & Windus.

8 Rituals and feasts

Food, art and spirituality

Introduction

The hunter-gatherers were the first of our ancestors to eat their meals cooked, as we do (Wrangham, 2009). Their cave paintings, the first evidence of the making of art by humans, reveal how they propitiated the spirits of the animals they killed for food. In these images, they recognize the gift of that sacrifice of life and show respect for the chance opportunity that made our species dominant. Their precariousness of survival was coped with by turning to some greater whole that could be trusted to provide the necessities for life, whether this was the forest itself, or the beach, or the beginnings of some kind of deity, 'gods whose existence would explain the inexplicable . . . friendly deities whose worship brought food in abundance' (Tannahill, 1973, p. 44). The making of image and story and song, and the knowing of sacredness all came from the desire to survive, and survival has, and always will, be about food.

I knew this book would cover a lot of ground and that if I were to comment on every aspect of food in our lives, which was my original aim, it might be difficult to avoid many disjointed 'Food and. . .' sections. Presenting a narrative whole that was coherent, meaningful and connected to the mental health and wellbeing of humans seemed like it might be a challenge, particularly with this chapter. Yet, as I write it now, moving towards the end of the book, I see how the 'shopping list' of chapter contents that I gathered all those months ago, when I was writing the original proposal, has indeed become a 'story'. It has grown into an account of how we have made meaning for ourselves as humans in our shared experience of life. This making of meaning is one of the attributes that differentiates us from other species of animals. It is what makes us storytellers, artists and musicians, as well as requiring us to seek the divine through worship and making us reverential towards the mystery of life.

Without access to the expressive arts, and to the spiritual (however we define that for ourselves), I believe we become less than human. In my own work, I notice that a sign of when people are beginning to come back from significant burnout or trauma, they begin to be creative again, whether that is through drawing, singing, writing poetry, gardening or cooking, or even just through how they live their lives. As health practitioners, we may need to cultivate our own

DOI: 10.4324/9781003172161-9

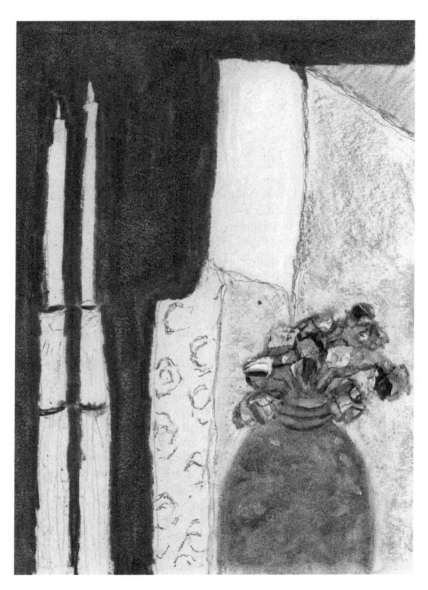

Hearth and heart

creative self-expression, so that we can be available to appreciate the ways in which our clients express theirs, and how that contributes to their mental health. Access to creativity is also very important for maintaining resilience in ourselves. This chapter offers some possible approaches that may make a useful contribution to both purposes.

Food and the arts

Our human preoccupation with food has provided us with subject matter for the expressive arts at both grass-roots level, and for master practitioners. Still life paintings of food hang on the walls of school classrooms and of museums. Our engagement with food is aesthetic and also visceral. Our senses and embodied processes fuel the connection between the arts and food and, without it our experience of life becomes diminished. People I have worked with who have described themselves as depressed talk about a lack of relish for what their life offers them. This bleak emptiness is both a symptom and a sign that there is likely to be a mental health issue involved.

Food and visual art

Written by Liz Hammond, Artist.

A history of art. Bite-sized, when there is so much to digest. . .

At my (mature student) art lessons, our end-of-term lunch tended to be communal, particularly at Christmas. I became aware – surprised, too at first – that the other students had taken such care with the food they brought, both in content and in presentation. I had always done so, thinking it was me being fussy, but here were other like-minded people to whom art and food were important parts of life and were treated accordingly.

It seemed to be the philosophy of the painting school that an interesting painting has complementary colours, contrasts and shapes in the way a plate of interesting food might: a stew, a salad, a buddha bowl. . . . Also, that if a drawing or painting was not quite right, it needed to be done again. It needed to be somehow aesthetically authentic. The painting – or the food -needed to be 'in conversation' with the viewer (or the eater in the case of food). It was also a celebration of both.

The history of art and food is one of both availability, and opportunity – that of showcasing the skill of the artist. Though this is a huge generalization, from the paintings executed before photography to, for example, Cezanne's 'new' way of painting fruit, food in paintings also served to illustrate the passage of life – the ripe fruit, or game hung for the table, will slowly deteriorate, wither and die as will we. Still Life is known, for example, as 'Nature Mort' in French. Foodstuffs are found as an adjunct to Egyptian tombs, to nourish the deceased in the afterlife. That is, after death. In the current society of the first world, ageing and death are often denied or unvalued. Wabi Sabi, the Japanese aesthetic, celebrates the imperfect, and the ageing process. It also celebrates the mysterious, the not-obviously-obvious in a painting, which one has to pause to look at, to wonder.

All very different for the sensual delight and palate of the maker, the eater, and particularly the viewer from the 'food porn' age of Instagram, and Masterchef's immediacy of image. However, food is made to be consumed and very often shared, a most important and significant human interaction. Perhaps the most famous 'meal' painting is Da Vinci's 'The Last Supper'; during the coronavirus pandemic, it was the family and friend-shared meals that were most missed – many were carried out via Zoom rather than not at all, as these shared meals represent so much, even virtually. Food and art are forever intertwined.

Food and literature/drama

One of the most pleasurable ways I know of connecting with a novel, or a play, or a film is to eat the same thing that their characters have been described as eating. I never went to boarding school but, after endless persuading, my mother let me stay up late one night for a midnight feast. It was probably only 10 o'clock, but it was dark. I had to eat the ginger cake and drink the lemonade with my mother, rather than with a group of exciting dorm-mates at 'Saint Clare's', but I remember vividly the excitement, and the uncomfortable feeling of food in my stomach when I should have been asleep. I read a lot of Enid Blyton as a child, and there were always picnics and tuck boxes and unexpected snacks that were described in great detail and to which I responded with enormous pleasure. I remember also that I would often eat while reading and that the doing of both was a consolation for me.

A bit later on, I watched, spellbound as Alan Bates ate a fig in the 1969 Ken Russell film 'Women in Love' which was based on the book by D.H. Lawrence. He quartered the fruit, cutting not quite to the base of it, so that it was possible to spread the segments and enclose them one-by-one with his mouth. I had never seen a fig and was not entirely sure they really existed, and I also did not quite understand the uneasy feeling I had from watching the scene. . .

There is also something about where it takes place that is connected with this desire to reproduce a literary meal. When I had to stay overnight in London for a work commitment, I decided to read Monica Ali's book while I was there, and to eat my dinner at Brick Lane. The book and the place together permitted me to enter a world different from my own. A similar principle applies with real people. When I was writing about Gertrude Stein and Alice B. Toklas for Chapter 6, I made a note of their address in the Rue de Fleurus and a resolution to visit it next time I'm in Paris. I want to see where Alice B. cooked fish for Picasso. On a previous trip to Paris, I went to the Café de Flore and drank Gin Fizz at 'l'heure de l'aperitif' in honour of Simone de Beauvoir.

I am not the only person who is intrigued by knowing about the food that characters eat. The dietary choices of the Sicilian detective Montalbano in the books by Andrea Camilleri have inspired many media posts from chefs, gastronomes and other commentators that are easily accessible by means of a Google search. What is it about humans that we want to eat like the people who fascinate us, even the fictitious ones? Perhaps writers know that the food each of us eats tells a lot about who we are, and where we come from, and want to use that detail to make their characters more real for the reader. By eating the same thing, or eating at the same time or place, we are somehow symbolically sharing the meal with the character.

Maybe it also has to do with the connection between ritual and story that is such a feature of organized religion. There is a deep satisfaction in repeating actions that have significance, and we recognize the power of that repetition in our sacred and secular rituals. I return to this theme later in the chapter. For now, I only suggest that sharing in a literary banquet is a deeply satisfying practice that feeds and sustains the mental health of those of us who enjoy it.

Food as art

If art takes food and makes it into a meaningful depiction that reveals something about what it means to be human, then cooking presents food as a piece of art to consume, literally as well as visually. Presenting a dish to someone who is about to eat has its own conventions. Somehow, it is natural to assemble the plate according to the customs the society to which we belong adopts. It is usually about serving food in a particular style, and with care, rather than just heaping it on a plate. How it looks is as important as how it smells and tastes for piquing the appetite. The aesthetics of our food traditions create connections between us and our societies and families, which help build the sense of identity and belonging that is so important for mental health and also for societal cohesion.

How food looks has become a preoccupation for those who like to post photographs of their meals on Instagram, or other social media platforms. It is common now to reach for a smartphone before raising a knife and fork. Food has become a significant part of what we currently tend to call 'lifestyle'. Sharing our lives (lifestyles?) on social media has become part of the way we socialize. What does it say about a person if they eat beautiful looking food at every meal? Well, it would depend on who is looking and in what circumstances. Maybe one reaction would be envy, or sceptical amusement at the display of ego, or maybe just acceptance that beautiful food can be available to all of us as a human right. Participating in society is essential for mental health, which is why social injustice caused by poverty, which can lead to the deprivation of food and everything connected with it, things like worth, belonging, choice and pleasure, is so devastating for those who suffer it.

Food writing has become a significant genre in recent years, and part of mainstream culture in the west. The characteristic that defines it is the emphasis on senses and the body. Finding the exact words to define a flavour and serving them up appetizingly on the page attracts readers, even though they may never actually make the dish that is being described. Besides books, food-related culture includes television series, festivals, talks and demonstrations. During the pandemic, cookery classes over Zoom became widely available, an idea that was new to me up until that time. Shared culture is like a conversation in which we all participate, one which has the power to shape the society in which we live. Often the conversation is about politics, current events or sport, as well as being about literature and the arts. Making food part of the conversation may help us to change our attitude to it and, hopefully, move away from the practices around it that are currently detrimental for us. Contributing to the way society evolves is an important part of being human and, without it, both the individual and society are diminished. As health professionals, we see the negative effects feelings of exclusion have on the mental health of our clients.

If fine art is different from art as an everyday creative expression, then restaurants are the equivalent of it in the food world. Those of us that can, or decide to, afford it can eat at legendary establishments run by icons of the food world. I well remember being at Padstow many years ago, before Rick Stein became famous, but still being thrilled when he came out into the restaurant towards the end of the evening to receive the smiles and applause that we diners showered on him. Almost like the celebrant of a religious service, he had acted as the inspired initiator of the shared experience and was acknowledged for it by the satiated participants. I have not been present at many such events but, when I am, they stay with me. Like an opera or a play, the experience transcends that of the everyday. This kind of taste of the numinous edges on to the spiritual and I develop the theme in later sections. If a visit to a grand restaurant is a high-end food experience, then meals at home are the everyday alternative. Of course, both are needed for a meaningful life and I pick this theme up too, later on.

Food and sex

I was taught by nuns at school, before the contraceptive pill became generally available, and when sex happened in the context of marriage and became shameful outside it, particularly for women. I think for boys and men too, although in a slighter way because they had a chance to distance themselves from the possible outcome in a way that girls and women could not. Nevertheless, there was still a lot of pressure for couples to marry if there was a child on the way, however unsuitable or unhappy the match.

In this environment, we studied Keats' poem 'The Eve of Saint Agnes'. This is an ambiguous story of a rape (there was no consent) and an abduction, presented as a romantic, swashbuckling tale. I suppose it got past the nuns because of the saint's name in the title. Agnes was one of the, what are called 'virgin martyrs', young women who choose death rather than defilement. For the lovers in the poem, after sex there was feasting and I was seduced by the images and language used to describe the food, the colour, abundance and fragrance of it. So, the connection between delicious food and delightful sex was established for me early in my life through knowing this poem, although it was quite a while before I experienced them together for myself.

The association between food and sex is used suggestively in visual art. Edouard Manet's portrait of 'The Street Singer' is the image of a woman going about her business in an everyday, slightly distracted manner. She is alone, fully clothed and in public. Yet she is carrying a bag of cherries, the brown paper parcel is grasped firmly in one arm, while the other hand raises a small bunch of the shiny fruit absent-mindedly to her lips. The portrait is of 'Victorine Meurent, who was Manet's favourite model up to 1875' (Malaguzzi, 2008, p. 246). Is it the image of the cherries themselves that is sexy? Or is it that they are being consumed in pleasurable profusion, heedless of the observer? Or anything else? I suppose, as always, it depends on who else is looking and under what circumstances. . .

Eating and sex are so connected in our experience of being human because both are instances of our meeting needs by reaching out into the world around us. I explored this dynamic earlier, in Chapter 4. Contacting the environment in the holistic way I described there involves body sensation, emotion and intellect. No wonder artists and writers use the association between food and sex to grab our attention. The need that is met by these stories and artistic representations is more emotional than purely physical, although all the aspects of our selves are connected and responsive to the experience. Some meaning is revealed for us about the universality of the human condition, and we find it profoundly satisfying. Nourishing every aspect of ourselves as humans, including this appetite for meaning making, keeps us mentally, emotionally and physically healthy.

Food and sex are so connected because each evokes a kind of eros. I have been trying to think of a way of defining my use of the word eros in this context and what I have come up with is to call it the thrill of being alive. By that I mean an experience that is heightened, just dangerous enough to be exciting while still being essentially safe, experienced in the body and, most importantly, the outcome of a kind of vital connection. This can happen during encounters in other contexts too.

I once had the opportunity to visit a person who had become something of a legend among those who knew him, recognized for his expertise and devotion to good cheese. I stepped out of a warm, Italian morning into the cool, lactic environment of his shop and there he was. Of course, his was a large presence, and he welcomed me while standing resplendently between his two female assistants, all of them covered in crisp, pristine white linen. I loved tasting and buying the cheese, but the memory that stays most vividly with me is of the cheesemonger explaining how, by talking about food, it was possible to enjoy it twice, and without double the calories. I laughed, and responded that, by writing about food, it was possible to enjoy it three times, still without the calories. . . . We spoke a mixture of Italian and English between us, according to the level of ability each of us had with the other's language. The shop is no longer there. The man who loved cheese decided to retire and concentrate on feeding himself rather than feeding his customers. But I still have the story. . . . We never so much as touched the other's hand, yet my memory is of an encounter that was ripe with eros. An experience such as this is possible whilst remaining fully clothed, but it is still intense and exciting. Access to this kind of heightened feeling is one of the fundamental aspects of being human. Each experience of it makes a contribution to the quality of our mental health. Lack of it leaves us bored and bleak.

Food porn is an expression that has come into common usage in recent time. Like regular pornography, food porn is about depictions of the experience, rather than the thing itself. As with great art, it involves pictures of food, which made me wonder what characterizes an image as food porn, what makes it different from the experience of looking at the Manet portrait, which did not seem to me to be pornographic? I realized that pornography does not involve eros, it is not relational.

The observer is detached rather than emotionally caught up in the experience. The image becomes objectified, something disposable, just there to be consumed, rather than a subject with which to create engagement. This reminds me of the discussions in previous chapters about current attitudes to food in western society. We must devour, digest and assimilate food with our bodies, just as we become one with another person during sex. Maybe value and respect are what makes the difference between eros and pornography in either context. Understanding the distinction helps us as health professionals to support our clients in making choices that are more truly nourishing for their mental and physical health.

Food as medicine

Food is medicine. Some health professions are devoted to healing people when they are sick, and traditional and modern approaches to mental and physical health use specific plants as medications. For example, aspirin, derived from willow bark, is freely available at chemists, supermarkets and corner-shops as a remedy for everyday ailments. Diseases of the heart are treated using foxgloves through the medication digoxin, and opiates (made from poppies) are commonly used in pain relief. These medicinal plants are not generally recognized as food although, as produce of the natural world they may be affected by the same issues of soil sustainability and land use associated with food plants.

Other professions are devoted to helping people choose diets that will keep them well: dietitians, nutritionists and others, and the first part of this book is all about how our choice of diet can affect our mental and physical health and wellbeing. There are also traditional systems that offer a wholistic approach to diet and health. The Ayurvedic approach is associated with thousands of years of such wisdom. I was introduced to this system about 30 years ago when I began to learn Transcendental Meditation. Someone at the centre told me that an Ayurvedic doctor was in the area and available for consultations. She had to explain to me that he was fully trained and qualified in western medicine, and also in the Ayurvedic approach. I kind of went along with her enthusiasm and being naturally curious, I booked a session. In it, we mostly talked about my experience of life and my diet, which I knew at the time was not a particularly healthy one. He would have noticed how overweight I was, firstly because it was quite obvious and also because the Ayurvedic method includes identifying body types, which determine the kind of diet that best suits each. There are three different categories, called 'doshas': vata, pitta and kapha. We all have a balance of each of them although one is often predominant. At first glance, I may have seemed like a kapha type, large and slow. But, he told me, I was more likely to fall into the pitta category (medium frame, intelligent) or maybe even vata (small frame and creative). Really? Me? I remember feeling sad for the light, swift self within me that was never revealed. I came away from the consultation with recommendations for dietary change, and the recognition of a new potential within myself. While the dietary change did not really stick at that time, I took up yoga and, through it, found out more about the Ayurvedic system, which is a comprehensive one. As well as different foods, particular times of day and seasons are associated with the doshas. While I am by no means expert, understanding how an individual's diet can link with the elemental energetic nature of the wider whole offers me a new perspective. This glimpse of the fundamental unity of being feeds my spiritual nature as much as the appropriate diet for my body feeds my physical nature. To be truly healthy, I believe humans need to nourish all the aspects of ourselves.

Artemisia is a herb I've seen growing in the wild in Italy. It is also one of the ingredients in the bottle of vermouth I have on the top shelf of one of my kitchen storage cabinets for when I want to make a negroni sbagliato. This is a version of the classic negroni cocktail, which is a blend of vermouth, Campari and gin. The sbagliato involves using prosecco rather than gin. The word means 'mistaken' in English, although I much prefer that version to the classic negroni. I'm not sure how possible it is to pick up a bottle of prosecco and mistake it for gin, but I am appreciative of the consequences of the accident. See the 'Food Note' at the end of the chapter if you want to know how I make it. The name reminds me of the seventeenth-century Italian artist, Artemisia Gentileschi, one of the very few women artists to be recognized for their masterpieces over the centuries.

Food and superstition

Every morning, as my porridge is warming on the stove, I take my wooden spoon and stir it. But only one way, only clockwise. Sometime so long ago that I cannot even remember when, someone told me, I cannot remember who, that stirring anti-clockwise allows the devil into the porridge. This is what superstition is, a veiled whisper without rational sense, yet suffused with echoes of ancient wisdom. I don't really believe in it, but why take the risk. . . . Every culture has their own food superstitions. A very common one in the UK involves salt. If any is spilled, then throwing a pinch over the left shoulder is a way of avoiding bad luck. As a child, I was always intrigued that there were two possible ways of accessing a boiled egg: slicing off the top in one piece or shattering the shell around the tip and picking away the shards. Superstition says that the little shell cup produced by the first method can be used as a boat for the devil. I do cut off the tops of my boiled eggs to open them these days, but I notice that I try and shatter the shell when I put it in the food recycling bin.

Folk tales are often seen as mundane versions of mythology, so maybe superstitions about food are an everyday reminder of the links between food and religion, which are widespread and rich.

Food and religion

Formal religions

Counted among the goddesses in ancient Greece is Hestia, goddess of both hearth and altar. These two realms may seem a strange combination at first, and yet the connections become clear with some consideration. Both hearth and altar involve fire: the fireside where families gather and the flame under the cooking pot and also the candles and lamps of worshippers. As well as being the protector of the domestic hearth, she is also, guardian of the community flame which symbolized the coherence and continuity of the state. To worship Hestia was to recognize the place of the household within the state. Mythology and religion reveal the significance of food, shelter and community from time out of mind. Sacred images and sounds evoke the meaning of this connection.

In ancient Greece, the famous 'Mysteries of Eleusis' were fertility rites, secret rituals attempting to ensure a bountiful harvest. Again, food, survival and religion were seen to be inseparable. The place of food in religious practice is still evident today. Christians have Holy Communion, the consecration of the bread and wine so that it becomes the body and blood of Christ. For Roman Catholics, 'transubstantiation' (transformation) happens as the priest speaks an account of 'The Last Supper', the Passover meal that Christ shared with his followers on the evening before his arrest and eventual crucifixion. The moment in the story when Christ blesses the bread and passes it around the table is when wafers on the altar in the local church take on a different nature.

The original last supper was a meal held in celebration of a previous holy event, which has its own story. The Israelites had come into Egypt and had eventually become slaves there. They wanted to return to the promised land, but the Egyptians would not let them go. After many attempts to persuade them, as a final inducement, God was to send the angel of death to kill the first born in every family. The Israelites were told to mark their doorsteps with the blood of a lamb, so that their households would be passed over (hence the name Passover). Afterwards, devastated with grief, the Egyptians final let the Israelites go, and their long journey through the desert, led by Moses, began. Food writer Claudia Roden observes that 'Every cuisine tells a story. Jewish food tells the story of an uprooted, migrating people and their vanished worlds. It lives in people's minds and has been kept alive because of what it evokes and represents' (1996, p. 3).

Food-related practices are part of the Islamic faith too, and so tell their own story. Certain foods, like pork are forbidden, as is alcohol. The fast of Ramadan, when no food or drink is taken between sunrise and sunset, is an important aspect of the faith, and there are teachings that emphasize the need for balance and moderation in food and drink intake, and general care of the body.

The Sikhs have their own stories and religious practices. Guru Nanak was the son of a wealthy landowner but showed no sign of wanting to follow his father into farming. In an attempt to find a profitable path for his son to follow, the father decided to give him 20 rupees and send him off to start his own business. Soon after he set out, Nanak came to a village where the people were sick and starving. He used his 20 rupees to buy food and clothing for them from another village. When his father challenged Nanak about what seemed in his eyes to be squandering the money, Nanak said that indeed he had made a 'True Bargain'. Helping the needy became enshrined in Sikhism, and their temples, even the Golden Temple at Amritsar became community kitchens as well as places of worship.

Maybe food is such an important element of so many religions because, again, it is essential for survival. It may also be the focus for rituals or customs that help to define a particular group of people and create cohesion around the traditions they share. For those that do adhere to a particular faith, it can be an important aspect of who they are and relevant, essential even, for maintaining mental health.

Even though many people do not actively practise a religion these days, the resonances of religious practices still have significance.

Secular feasts: to gather together

When the sacred also infuses the ordinary and everyday it brings a sheen to existence. The close involvement between food and the spiritual makes the kitchen a natural focus for attitudes and practices that enhance every-day life. Mealtimes can become secular rituals, and the dining table can be something akin to an altar as people gather around it, coming together to share an experience of sustenance, pleasure and connection. I know that, in real life, often meals can be hasty necessities, taken while the attention is elsewhere, but the availability of three opportunities a day to gather, reflect and become present means that there are plenty of possibilities for accessing what I like to call the numinous.

The word comes from numen, a Latin expression describing a divine presence or spirit. Sometimes people use the word grace to describe a similar quality. My experience is that the numinous is always there when we turn to find it. Turning towards something that is greater than we are or that transcends our everyday experience, seems always to have been part of the human condition and we may access it through a beautiful (though not necessarily pretty) painting, a poem or story, a song or a piece of music as well as through ritual or prayer.

I mentioned the neo-lithic cave paintings earlier, and we still hear the echoes of past civilizations in stories of gods and goddesses, heroes and heroines, monsters and subterranean kingdoms. We can find traces of the fairy folk, saints and hermits, in place names and landscape features like 'fairy' mounds and holy wells. Some people find a connection to the spiritual sphere through organized religion, others find it through meditation, or being in nature, or, of course, through food. It is a fundamental part of being human and therefore necessary for our mental health.

The sacred kitchen

Here are some ways of making the preparation and participation involved with food more mindful:

- Let kitchen routines become secular rituals by carrying out activities like preparing vegetables, cooking and clearing up, with the intention of making them meaningful actions. Intention is very powerful and can allow us to access the universal in the particular.
- Light candles. At one time, when I began cooking a meal, I would set a tea-light in front of a small triptych depicting a radiant woman. I think the image was meant to be of the Virgin Mary, but for me she depicted a universal principle of transcendence. Now, I have a chubby pillar candle in the centre of my dining table, which I light when I set the places for a meal, even at breakfast.

- Arrange flowers or branches and leaves, depending on the time of year, and place them around the home.
- Celebrate family festivals. In my family those would be Christmas, Easter and birthdays. You may have other traditions, in accordance with your own background. Be mindful of how these repeated rituals have the possibility of knitting together families and society. Tell the stories of previous celebrations, share memories of grandparents or other relatives who are no longer alive. Sing the songs.
- Use the power of shared meals to bring communities together. In Britain, the tradition is for street parties. Other kinds of shared meals might involve each person or family bringing a dish of food to share among everyone. These kinds of shared meals are common when people have been undergoing some kind of learning activity together and are powerful celebratory markers. Work teams often go out together for meals at Christmas, or to celebrate particular shared achievements.
- Many people give thanks for the bounty of a meal by saying a form of words. These words could be called a prayer, if that fits the person's belief system. They are also sometimes called a 'grace'. Pausing to acknowledge the significance that surrounds the eating of a meal; having access to food because the harvest has been successful, owning sufficient resources to be able to obtain it and a safe place in which to eat it, maybe surrounded by a group of people we care about, and who care about us. A simple meal symbolizes fulfilment of many of the deepest needs we have as humans and, taking time to remember this brings enormous satisfaction and a sense of gratitude.

Undertaking these, or other small actions can transcend the experience of the everyday and reveal a glimpse what we might call the divine, whether or not it is connected with a particular deity or belief system. Bringing a sense of meaning and connection, they contribute towards meeting the soul-needs that are so much part of what makes us human. Tying fulfilment of these needs with food, offers three chances a day for meditative moments that sustain us spiritually while our bodies, minds and emotions are sustained by the nourishment and pleasure of eating a meal. Health practitioners are likely to have opportunities to witness the place of the spiritual in the lives of the people with whom we work. Often, their beliefs or practices may be different to our own but, reflecting on the shared human needs underlying them may help us work with others more effectively, and also increase our own resources.

Death

'Death is outside life but it alters it: it leaves a hole in the fabric of things that those who are left behind try to repair. Perhaps it is because of this that we are minded to feast at funerals' (Vickers, 2000, p. 3). At the very end, when death arrives to disrupt the assumption that all will go on as it did before, food still has its place.

Legendary food writer M.F.K. Fisher wrote about the imminent death of her lover. 'We were very live ghosts, and drank and ate and saw and felt and made love better than ever before, with an intensity that seemed to detach us utterly from life' (Fisher, 2017, p. 253). They were travelling in Europe at the time, in 1939, just before the Second World War began. How the outside world must have reflected the intimate, time-limited one shared by the lovers then.

Flavours become more poignant with the prospect of death, or loss; experience is heightened. The proximity of death makes being alive more vital. We forget this attribute of being for most of the time, until death comes close, whether it is our own, or that of someone important to us. How each of us faces the prospect of death tells a lot about our philosophy of life, I believe. While death does not yet lurk directly behind the door for me, I am closer to it now than I am to birth. Those two great bookends, birth and death, frame our lives. The still life paintings of food are there to remind us of it, so are the stories of other people's deaths and losses that show us how we might behave when the unthinkable up to that very moment happens to us. If we look to food, maybe it is for reassurance of our own aliveness and the continuing cycle of life. Our preparedness to encounter death is an important contribution to mental health. We do not talk about death much in our society. It has been a great unmentionable, so we do not know what to say when we meet someone we know who is suffering, whether from having to come to terms with the proximity of their own death, or from the loss of someone essential in their lives. Thinking and talking about death reminds us that it is part of our shared humanity. Maybe, in order to be able to do that, we find comfort in the partaking of food.

Chapter summary

The miracle of survival as a species has inspired humans to produce great works of art, poetry and music. We know our selves through the stories we tell, whether we categorize them as mythology, history, literature, news or conversation. Being conscious of our selves, in the way that other animals are not, we look for something 'other' to bring illumination and meaning into our struggle and bafflement. We can find this in spiritual practice, and also in the everyday rituals of being, particularly those related to food. Being able to create this connection to the numinous is essential for our mental health. Helping others to find it may be a significant part of our roles as health professionals in some contexts.

Activities

8.1 Individual

Write for ten minutes exploring the rituals around food that are meaningful for you. Leave what you have written unread for at least one day, then return and re-read it. Design and perform a ritual based on what you have written. This could be anything that has meaning for you.

8.2 With one other person

Find a family member and talk about what food means in your family, the traditions you have around food, and the emotional quality of your family's particular relationship with it. How does that connect to the way births, marriages and deaths are celebrated?

8.3 Group Activity

The group here could be of family members, work colleagues or clients. It could also be an individual activity that relates to a group. Consider the group on which you are focusing (family, workplace, community or other context). What are the commonalities and differences in the food traditions and attitudes present in the group? How do they affect the smooth-running of the group?

Personal reflection

On Food as Communion
Sharon Usher, Group Facilitator and Clown

Having been born and raised a Roman Catholic the embodied symbolism of ingestion as something more than a biological necessity has been present from day one. You could say I took it in with my mother's milk. I still recall the thrill and feeling of 'specialness' of preparing for, and then actually participating in, my First Holy Communion. My mother sewed a white broderie anglaise dress for me and I wore her wedding veil. I knew that I was to receive the 'Body of Christ' into my own body and that this was significant. And very holy indeed. I remember the practice hosts we were given beforehand. We were told not to chew, but to reverently allow the host to dissolve in our mouths whilst praying like billyoh.

I think this early experience of symbolism of ingestion has stayed with me. My childhood as a member of an extended family of Irish Catholics meant that as well as the Body of Christ that we all received every Sunday, we shared countless meals around many a makeshift extended table. I remember that the wallpaper pasting table plus the collapsible green baize card table were regularly called into service. The sharing of food and, it has to be said, far more wine than was strictly necessary, has been central to my sense of belonging.

This was underlined for me when I joined an inclusive spiritual community in my forties. By then I had left the Catholic Church and become a fully paid-up spiritual seeker outside of any formalised religion. However, I found, again, that shared food was important in more ways than simply providing for the energy needs of the body. The community was open to people of all faiths and none, and there was no designated spiritual practice apart from shared silence within which people did their own thing. And shared meals were central. They were not the formalised ritual of Catholic Communion but there was a ritualistic element to them that seemed to affect the collective life for the better. When we cooked, we did so with conscious attention and love. We attended to the beauty of the food in simple ways, nasturtium flowers with the salad, a sprinkle of paprika on the home-made hummus. And we held hands around the table and were silent before eating. These small and regular rituals seemed to build up the atmosphere of welcome in the community and we would regularly get what seemed like out of proportion com-pliments from visitors and guests for what was essentially simple vegetarian food cooked by amateurs. In this respect the meals were a form of agape, or love feast, which is defined as a communal meal shared amongst Christians. I wasn't sitting there in my white dress and veil, and rarely around that table did anyone say they were a Christian, but I recognised the deep feeling of nourishment beyond food. It was everyday, it was ordinary, it was without pompous ceremony or specialness. And holy.

Food note

Taste has its own set of categories. We recognize five distinct types of flavour: sweet, sour, bitter, salty and umami. The taste buds that activate in response to each of these different flavours are grouped together in various areas of the tongue. Salty is at the very tip, handy for a quick sample of a bag of crisps or a spoonful of soup. Right behind, and very accessible, come the detectors for sweet, maybe the favourite of the flavours for many of us, because the food that is available to us these days often has a lot of sugar in it. Further towards the back, and on each side, are the areas for detecting sour. Sometimes I can feel them tingle as a spritz of lemon juice hits them. In between, lies the area connected with the flavour called umami. This flavour seems rather exotic to me, probably because it is a Japanese word. It means savoury and that being the case, my first association is with miso soup and soy sauce, but it is also used to describe the flavour of meat generally, sardines, tomatoes and mushrooms. It is a relative newcomer to the pantheon of flavour, having been recognized and adopted in 1985. To the average tongue, it might comprise a hotch-potch of flavours not covered elsewhere, but the logic behind its adoption is that it is associated with a particular amino acid L-glutamate. Monosodium glutamate (MSG) is a familiar flavouring in oriental cuisine.

The very back of the tongue is where we sense bitterness. I came to value the taste of bitter in Sicily. The cliché is to connect Italy with 'La Dolce Vita' (the sweet life) but poverty, frugality and other societal challenges bring bitter-ness to the experience too. 'Amaro' is a word I came to know well as I learned about Sicilian food culture. I gathered and tasted the bitter greens that grow wild there in Spring and even now, back in Wales, every February, when the new grass comes at Imbolc (the early Spring Celtic festival celebrated around 2nd February) my body craves for this bitterness. I find it in dandelion leaves, sourcing them from areas with no risk of animal urine, and washing and dry-ing them carefully before stir-frying gently in (Sicilian) olive oil). Sometimes, in Farmer's Markets, I can find the larger, more substantial leaves that Italians call 'cicoria' (chick -or-reeyah) that are just like monster dandelion leaves and nothing like the bulbs of paler, fatter leaves that greengrocers here seem to call chicory, although those are bitter too. I've discovered a supplier for cicoria seeds, so I can grow my own. There is a link to information about a film that explores 'amaro' in the resources section.

My other favourite way of enjoying bitter is through the drink called 'negroni sbagliato' (discussed previously). I usually make this in a large jug that I fill with ice before sloshing in a glug of vermouth and a glug of Campari and topping up with prosecco. I pour into small, chunky tumblers allowing a few cubes of ice to drop in each glass, and add a small segment of orange, just for a tiny hint of sweet that highlights the bitter drink. The amount of orange that complements the glasses I use is about one sixth of a slice. Imagine the disk of an orange with a small hole in the middle where the segments meet, is a birthday cake and divide it into six segments with a sharp knife.

Because I usually mix it 'freehand', I was unsure about the proportions of the ingredients and I had to do some research. I discovered that I like one part vermouth, one part Campari and six parts prosecco. The 'part' here can be a spoon of an appropriate size, or a measure. I have a glass measure and I poured into it 10 millilitres of vermouth, 10 of Campari and then filled up to the 80 mark with prosecco. This is a strong drink, so not many are required at a time in order to feel celebratory. I am also aware that I have previously been describing the negative effects of alcohol on the body and brain, so maybe moderation is a good thing here. Perhaps doing what the Italians do and having something to eat with an alcoholic drink is a helpful strategy. In Britain, the obvious thing would be a bowl of crisps but, sometimes a dish of olives, black or green, and some breadsticks are a welcome alternative. Cubes of cheese or vegetarian pâté and maybe slices of salami are also good on more elaborate occasions. A drink that is more bitter and less potent is Campari and soda water (one part Campari and six parts soda with a slice of lemon suits my taste). A non-alcoholic voyage into bitter could involve equal parts of blood-orange juice and fizzy bitter lemon drink.

We need contrast for heightening experience. This is as true of flavours as it is of feelings. We must have the bitter in order to really appreciate the sweet, just as having challenges in our lives makes ease more enjoyable. The ability to embrace all the possibilities of interaction with the world is part of being human and an important contribution to mental health.

References

Fisher, M.F.K. (2017) *The gastronomical me*. London: Daunt Books (first published in 1943 by Duell, Sloan and Pearce, New York).

Malaguzzi, S. (2008) *Food and feasting in art* (trans. Phillips, B.). Los Angeles: J. Paul Getty Museum.

Roden, C. (1996) *The book of Jewish food*. London: Penguin Books.

Tannahill, R. (1973) *Food in history*. London: Eyre Methuen.

Vickers, S. (2000) *Miss Garnet's angel*. London: HarperCollins.

Wrangham, R. (2009) *Catching fire*. London: Profile Books.

9 Digestif

Satisfaction and integration

Introduction

This final chapter brings together the different aspects of food and mental health and seeks to identify the conditions that need to be in place for human beings to thrive. Dealing with difference and being able to withstand and resolve conflict are important contributory factors for maintaining individual and societal mental health, and also for helping us to address the issues of inequality, food insecurity and threats to the natural environment that challenge us. Some observations around the nature of conflict in families, neighbourhoods and other organizations are offered in relation to that end.

While health professionals are encouraged to integrate the information and ideas offered in the book into their practice, they are also invited to pay attention to their own competence for working with the issues, and understand where the limits are in particular situations. Suggestions of ways of accomplishing this are outlined. A case study is offered for how competence might be demonstrated. A final 'Personal Reflection' comes from a contributor and is a description of how a family's relationship with food used to look and could look again.

Conditions for mental health

'Health . . . is not something that is revealed by investigation but rather manifests itself by the virtue of escaping our attention' (Heaton, 1998, p. 38). Yet this has been a book about food and mental health. Over the various chapters I have considered different aspects of what it means to be human, and how food is a constant factor in the way our lives unfold. At this point, it seems appropriate to gather together the various constituents into a whole and define the conditions that need to be in place for human beings to experience what it means to be healthy.

Is this a menu or a recipe? I think it has to be both. With a menu, we can choose our favourite items from the list. With a recipe, we have to create the meal ourselves from the ingredients we have. In life, as in the kitchen, what you have is not as important as how you use it. The ability to make something meaningful from the life experiences we have is equivalent to the ability to use what is available in

DOI: 10.4324/9781003172161-10

fridge and cupboards to create a plate of wholesome, tasty, satisfying food. I think both are essential skills.

Putting together this list, I notice that a lot of the things we need for mental health are actually physical, and that a lot of them come from the environment in which we live, rather than from the ways we express our selves in the world. 'Humans are tuned for relationship. The eyes, the skin, the tongue, ears and nostrils- all are gates where our body receives the nourishment of otherness' (Abram, 1997, p. ix). Again and again in the book, I have come back to the significance of our interconnectedness with each other and with the world in which we live, and here I am again, maybe for the last time.

Conditions for mental health

Context:

> Secure shelter in a clean environment
> Access to pure water
> Sufficient food of appropriate nutritional quality
> Family and Community
> Respect for bodily and psychological integrity

Self:

> Keen senses – touch, taste, smell, sight, hearing
> Access to and appropriate expression of full emotional range
> Ability to focus thought and still the mind
> Capacity to encounter challenges with courage and resilience
> Spiritual and creative expression

Interpersonal:

> Ability to contribute to joint problem solving with others
> Awareness of the human tendency to treat people who are not like us
> differently from those who are
> Acknowledgement of injustice
> Capacity for forgiveness, remorse and reconciliation
> Capability to withstand and resolve conflict

I have touched on most of these conditions over the course of the book, but one of them is particularly important for creating a just and sustainable future and needs to be explored as the book comes to an end. It is the capability to withstand and resolve conflict.

Difference and conflict

People are different and have different views about how things 'should' be, so conflict and even aggression are not far beneath the surface in a shared life space (see Chapter 6). The way groups organize around conflict situations influences participants' experience, and also how effectively group and individual needs can be met within them. Sometimes conflict is handled informally while other conflict situations seem to require structures to support the procedures.

Recognizing difference and having ways to resolve any conflicts are important in work environments. I include local and national governments and international structures and protocols as work environments in this context, as well as companies, churches and communities. Formal or informal processes for dealing with conflict often become part of the culture of an organization. It is possible to use difference positively. If two or more people, or groups, have seemingly opposing ideas, working through them, discovering more about the potential plusses and minuses of each, can often result in a synthesis that produces a solution that is much better than any of the original possibilities. Difference is also needed for creativity. A new and original solution or possibility emerges from a whole situation, rather than from the imagination of an individual. The 'disruptors', like Facebook, Amazon, Netflix etc., are those that can respond to the possibilities of developing technology and to the developing wants and needs of society, and who try out their ideas often enough to happen to be lucky once. The benefits of difference make it important for there to be diversity among decision-makers and innovators, and it is particularly valuable if it reflects the diversity of the community the organization serves. When conflict cannot be resolved productively, whether it is between individuals within the organization, or between management and employees, within or between governments, or in international disputes, policies and procedures for mediation, discipline or grievance are usually in place. When they fail, then the only recourse is to war, whether that is actual armed conflicts or bitter disputes, which are deadly and destructive for all involved.

Conflicts arise in the more intimate areas of our life space too. Certainly, it is present in families, although there the ties are different. Confrontation can be more direct because the fall-out is powerful and immediate, and there is a lot of investment in the outcome, as well as relatively easy access between the parties involved because they live together. In families there is more opportunity for dealing with issues through discussion and some kind of compromise or accommodation, although that is not always possible. In my observation, very often people just adjust to how things are – accept what is 'familiar'. Only when things go seriously wrong do they examine the dynamics of love and belonging, power, hatred and rejection, give and take, that provide each family with its own unique flavour. At some point, GPs or schoolteachers may be consulted, relationship counselling may be sought, or lawyers involved.

Neighbourhoods are shared fields. Living in proximity to other households means that the choices made by one often have an impact on the others. Noise, car-parking and overhanging trees are some of the areas in which conflict can occur. Much of the day-to-day impact is self-managed by those involved, with the local council being the arbiter of final resort. I had some work done at the back of my house and the contractor left unused materials behind, piled up near my garage door. I hadn't really noticed them, or how long they had been there, but the neighbour opposite definitely had. I received a letter from the local council notifying me that an (anonymous) neighbour had complained and demanding that the materials be removed within a certain deadline. I passed the letter on to the contractor and he took them away, so that was a relatively straightforward resolution. Others are not so easily resolvable, where there are ongoing boundary disputes for example.

This intimate kind of conflict resolution that takes place in families is less usual or possible when the house next door, or down the road is involved. Conflict with neighbours is potentially easier to ignore than when it is directly in a family because of this relative distance. There are societal structures like the police, solicitors and local and national government that respond to this kind of conflict. Structures are necessary when the people involved cannot, or do not resolve conflict for themselves. In some ways, deferring to a structure is easier as there is less emotional investment. We need structures that are fit for purpose. I believe that we also need the skills and opportunity to resolve conflict at a personal level, which means that we probably all need training in how to do it. Training and education for the kind of high-level personal skills we will all need to develop so that we can address the issues of inequality, food security and climate change we face could be part of a way forward.

Health practitioners and food

Limits to competence

Just as we regulate food intake according to appetite, but with a seasoning of knowledge and information, we make decisions about the limit of our remits as health professionals. This book is not attempting to make all of us into all-singing all-dancing experts around personal and societal relationships with food – that is an impossibly wide aspiration. Instead, it is about helping us know where our training and experience give us expertise, and when we need to refer on – to other trusted practitioners, or to books and websites that inform the decision-making capacity of our clients, and respect their autonomy.

How do we assess our competence? Korn (2016) suggests taking into account the legislative demands and structures that cover the areas in which we work. In my own previous book (Hughes, 2014), I talk about a framework of practitioner, client and context, which covers the training and experience of the practitioner, the nature and situation of the client and the context in which the work takes place, both physical and regulatory.

Supervision

In my profession, we all have access to supervision. For those who are unfamiliar with the concept, it involves meeting with a trusted senior practitioner at regular intervals for a specified time. With my caseload, 1 hour once a month meets the requirements of my accrediting organization (UK Council for Psychotherapy). Other accrediting bodies have different requirements.

To my own sessions I bring any difficulties I may be experiencing – clients I find particularly challenging because of their issues (or mine), when work seems to be stuck, or when it goes well. I also consult her about regulatory requirements, academic literature and general professional issues. She helped me integrate the knowledge I gained and preoccupations I experienced while I was writing this book into my therapeutic work with clients.

Case study – small family intervention

Written by Liz Hammond.

Here is an example of where a knowledge of the impact and meaning of activities related to food helped to resolve an issue swiftly and concretely.

'In the organizational setting where I was working, a young woman came to see me who had moved to the UK a few years previously. She was living in a two-bedroomed flat with her two children around 11 and 13. English was not her first language, but she explained to me that she felt she was somehow becoming distant from her children, whose father was also absent. Their behaviour had slightly deteriorated.

There are many unknown, and known, factors that might have influenced this situation. However, in talking at our first session, we drew together a plan of the interior of her flat. This prompted my question 'where do you eat your meals'? . . . .' on the sofa/armchair watching tv'.

'Do you have a table?' I asked. She did but it was the kind with an extendable flap, and it was pushed against the wall with two dining chairs either side also against the wall.

We discussed how the furniture might be moved, in a practical way, to enable space for the table to be pulled out, the two chairs used plus a stool, giving space for the three of them to sit and eat their meals there. We agreed to meet in two weeks, and she left saying she would try it. For the following session, she arrived in a different way – lighter, smiling – her whole demeanour had changed. She had immediately got the children involved in changing the furniture, and there perhaps surprisingly, had been little resistance to moving away from the comfy seats and the television to eat at the table. I had, as yet, no knowledge of their previous history of meals or indeed extended family. She recounted that it felt much more of a family unit, that they spoke to each other and connected more, 'like we used to'. So, our second session was also our last.

Whether or not I had intuited that before moving here, they had eaten together as a family, is unclear, as we had no further discussions where I might have discovered more about her history. However, since to most people in the world who have food, sharing it together is something very basic, it wasn't difficult to take a guess. The lack of this sharing together may well have consolidated the feelings about what had been lost by moving away from the 'old' home to a new one. Very brief systemic interventions don't always work so well, but this was such an example of a demonstration that 'how' we eat is as important, sometimes more so, than what we eat.

Chapter summary

It is possible for each of us to identify how mental health can be defined and how we can support it in our work with others. Sensitivity to the powerful influence of food in people's lives may make a contribution to that definition of mental health as a result of reading this book.

The way in which we handle conflict in our own lives and help our clients deal with it in theirs is significant.

Health professionals are required to attend to their personal and development and fitness to practice. Reflection on competence, particularly on where the limits to our own competence lie in a particular situation, is an important contribution to that process.

Activities

Please consider the following questions. This may involve thinking about them, meditating on them or making a piece of free-flowing, uncensored writing, similar to those in a personal journal.

9.1 Individual

Look at the list of 'Conditions for Mental Health' mentioned earlier. Taking each one in turn, write a few sentences about how it is expressed in your own life.

9.2 With one other person

Show what you have written and talk about it with one other trusted person.

9.3 Environmental

How might what you have learned be expressed in your work with clients? Do it.

Personal reflection

Food for thought

Written by Amanda Wood – Founder and Owner of The Micro Greengrocer (see Resources section)

> I grew up in the North East of England in the 1970's, the youngest of three children. We had a vibrant upbringing, with lots of activities provided by mum and dad, something I only recently appreciated while reflecting where my skills and interests originated. We were blessed with lots of performing, visual art and craft activities and with endless days helping in the garden allotment and greenhouse. We knew from a young age that we had the collective

skills not only to imagine but to make, create or grow almost anything. We were always able to put nutritious vegetables on the dinner table and fruit in our pies and puddings. I can remember, with all my senses, the colours, smells and textures of ceremoniously scrubbing potatoes clean; the taste of fresh peas while shelling them for one of mum's glorious Sunday roast dinners. When supermarkets started producing bags of washed potatoes, I think we lost something more important than just soil.

We had three good-sized gardens as we were on an end plot; interestingly shaped and well- established spaces, with lots of places to play. My childhood is packed full of memories of days inventing recipes and potions from the huge selection of flowers and herbs we had growing. Even now the smell of fresh basil is a trigger for the peaceful connection I have with this time.

Mum would batch cook pies and bakery items. The kitchen worktops would be filled with all sorts of delights that would duly be bagged up and stored in the chest freezer for rationing out over the weeks. We also had a family friend who was a pig farmer, a hard-hitting introduction to the reality of seeing where our meat was coming from. Needless to say, we ate a lot of pork. I suspect the important rationing skills that Mum employed were learnt from her mother during the Second World War and through the national recovery that lasted for years afterwards.

Although Mum had two – and sometimes three – jobs and Dad worked full-time as a telecommunications engineer, money must have been tight. This was probably why we practised a sort of self-sufficiency as a family. Mum was skilled at making food stretch more than the pennies, and we always had well balanced, delicious meals. There were times, unbeknown to us, when the money ran out. Mum with all her frugal creativity, would present us with what food was left. Mum could make egg and chips exciting, create an exotic 'Chinese' rice dish with spam and odd vegetables and used her creative enthusiasm to make everything a gourmet delight – and we loved it! I'm quite thankful that Mum didn't have to go through the hidden stress that would go with this façade too often.

Healthy eating habits and being involved with growing and preparing meals was embedded during these formative years. Mealtimes were also an important part of our upbringing, and this still features hugely in my life. Our mealtime would be the one time when all the family would come together each day. The table would be laid eagerly by myself or my hungry siblings. Table manners were of upmost importance: we would wait for everyone to be seated, before being told we could start dishing up our plates; however hungry we felt, we would never take more than we needed; we didn't talk a great deal during the meal as we were too focused on enjoying every mouthful. We knew table etiquette from a very early age, and when we finished our meal, we would always thank our mum and politely ask to leave the table.

I still make time for this mindful practice today. Having gratitude for being able to provide nutritious meals, and never overeating or wasting food means that left-over meals are saved and frozen or reinvented into another dish the following day.

Food note

Inequality, food security and climate change: these challenges have been identi-fied again and again over the course of the book. They test the mental health of all of us and require us to work together as global citizens. We face a dire prospect, but it can be a potentially transformational one too. There are already indications of a possible way forward. 'A replenished participation in the human collective, forging new forms of place-based community and planetary solidarity, along with a commitment to justice and the often exasperating work of politics' is one helpful suggestion (Abram, 2011, p. 9).

Naomi Klein observes:

> There are ways of preventing this grim future, or at least making it a lot less dire. But the catch is that these also involve changing everything. For us high consumers, it involves changing how we live, how our economies function, even the stories we tell about our place on earth.
>
> (2015, p. 4)

Everything changes. As health professionals, we witness the slow evolution of society that is taking place over time. Our role is to support people to remain healthy and resourceful in order to be able to make a contribution. This includes our selves. If you have come to the end after reading the whole book, then your willingness to engage and reflect has probably already made a contribution to the unfolding future. Emphasizing the positive, things each of us can do to arrive at where we want to be, serves mental health better than bemoaning the enormity of it all. We are well placed to witness and contribute to this unfolding. I wish us all well with the task of passing on a just and sustainable world to the next generations.

References

Abram, D. (1997) *The spell of the sensuous*. New York: Vintage Books.
Abram, D. (2011) *Becoming animal*. USA: Vintage Books.
Heaton, J. (1998) 'The enigma of health', *European Journal of Psychotherapy, Counsel-ling and Health*, 1(1), pp. 33–42.
Hughes, G. (2014) *Competence and self-care in counselling and psychotherapy*. Hove: Routledge.
Klein, N. (2015) *This changes everything*. UK: Penguin Random House.
Korn, L. (2016) *Nutrition essentials for mental health*. New York: Norton.

Appendix
Resources

There are many resources connected to food and mental health in books, articles, podcasts and websites. Here are some that have been valuable to me or recommended by colleagues.

Resources related to specific chapters

Chapter 3

Roots: factors underlying relationships with Food

Books:

Potatoes Not Prozac by Kathleen DesMaisons
In Defence of Food by Michael Pollan
First Bite: How We Learn to Eat by Bee Wilson
Mad Diet by Suzanne Lockhart
Spoon Fed by Tim Spector
The Food Mood Connection by Uma Naidoo
Understanding Your Eating: How to Eat and Not Worry about It.

Websites:

Julia Buckroyd Understanding your eating
www.understandingyoureating.co.uk
Links to academic articles on eating disorders:
www.kcl.ac.uk/people/professor-janet-treasure
www.kcl.ac.uk/people/ulrike-schmidt

Chapter 5

A World of Food: history and current situation

Books:

Two books by Carolyn Steel that have been invaluable for me for understanding the history of food, our current situation in relation to food production and distribution, and how a more sustainable, nourishing future might evolve:

'Hungry City' originally published by Vintage in 2009. I use the 2013 edition.
'Sitopia' published by Chatto & Windus in 2020. See: carolynsteel.com and
@carolynsteel.
For a description of the role of microorganisms in our bodies, and in the soil in which
our food is grown. Co-written by a professor of geomorphology (land forms)
and a biologist and environmental planner who are in a partner relationship
'The Hidden Half of Nature' by David R. Montgomery and Anne Biklé. Pub-
lished in 2016 by Norton.
Books with associated themes:
Eating Animals by Jonathan Safran Foer
Captive State by George Monbiot

Podcasts:

Engaging and informative discussion, hosted by Nathalie Nahai, with Tessa
Clarke, CEO and co-founder of Olio, a food-sharing app that enables neighbours to share any surpluses.
(olioex.com)
The Hive Podcast No.44 'Food, Sustainability and your Power to Change the World'

Websites:

WRAP – For addressing food waste issues
www.wrap.org.uk/about-us/about
UN on Food waste
www.fao.org/food-loss-and-food-waste/flw-data)#:~:text=One%2Dthird%20
of%20food%20produced,1.3%20billion%20tonnes%20per%20year
A plan for sustainable food production
www.foodsensewales.org.uk/pdf/FPACManifestoEnglish_091120.pdf
'Healthy Diets from Sustainable Food Systems':
EAT/Lancet Commission
https://eatforum.org/content/uploads/2019/07/EAT-Lancet_Commission_
Summary_Report.pdf

Chapter 6

Difference and Diversity

Websites:

Gordon Wheeler's speech at Budapest
www.youtube.com/watch?v=X-5ocN_0C14&list=PLkXcEt-KJO8K_
WLhsLmDIyIIzNA19hPzA&index=6
Vervaeke, John. 2020. *Awakening from the Meaning Crisis. Ep10. Consciousness.* www.youtube.com/watch?v=dRzm_wSR1RU

Chapter 7

Vital Virtual

Podcasts:

BBC Food Programme
Lab-grown meat 18th April 2021
Genome editing and the future of food 7th March 2021

Websites:

Complex systems
www.project-syndicate.org/commentary/green-from-the-grassroots?barrier=a
ccesspaylog

Chapter 8

Rituals and Feasts: food, art and spirituality

Podcasts:

From What If to What Next Episode 17 Hosted by Rob Hopkins
'What if indigenous wisdom could save the world?
Sherri Mitchell (Weh'na Ha'mu Kwasset) (USA) and Tyson Yunkaporta (Australia)
    share their ancestral wisdoms.,
Bitter
www.kickstarter.com/projects/amaro/amaro-the-bitter-taste-in-sicilian-food-culture

Chapter 9

Digestif: satisfaction and integration

An essay by contributor Amanda Wood about micronutrients and mental health:
https://drive.google.com/file/d/1sxqcr4L05Asi8U6WdK5agfazLlfmbXQ0/
    view?usp=sharing

General Related Topics

Books:

Much Depends on Dinner by Margaret Visser
The Circadian Code by Dr. Satchin Panda
BBC Sounds:
The Food Programme
30th August 2020 'Sitopia'

19th July 2020 'Food and Mood: how eating affects tour mental health'.
(many other general editions of the programme have relevance)
'Free Thinking' 2011 Susie Orbach
The Guardian articles:
Can food change your mood?
Dr Luisa Dillner. 17 Dec 2017
Food for thought . . . the smart way to better brain health
Lisa Mosconi, 13th October 2018
Poor diet link to riding cases of depression
Jo Revill, 5th January 2006

Websites:

COVID symptom App which is also powered by ZOE, the gut/diet research
    resource.
Plastic free living
www.onecommune.com/the-plastic-free-challenge-with-kate-nelson-free-5-day-
    pass-sign-up?__s=yxx0h1bwexp61gq8m1cb&utm_source=drip&utm_
    medium=email&utm_campaign=The+Pandemic+of+Plastic – Take+back+
    your+health%2C+Helen

Index

administrative staff, working from home 136–7
adrenalin 9, 42
affluence 36, 83, 100, 112–13, 124
age 101–2
aggression, in Gestalt 55–6
Agricultural Revolution 83
agriculture 25, 80, 123; *see also* farming
alcohol 101–2; food with 156; and inflammation 9
Alexa 122, 130
Ali, Monica 144
alkalinity 35
Alzheimer's disease 8, 36, 101
'amaro' 155–6
amino acids 7, 21, 155
anger 39, 42, 45–7, 52
anorexia 32–3, 38
antibiotics 9, 20
anxiety: in case studies 44–5; and diet 8, 23–4; social roots of 124; and stress 122
art: culinary 12; expressive 141, 143; and food 11–12, 143–6
artemisia 149
arthritis 40, 101
asthma 101
Attenborough, David 92
austerity 85
autism 8, 36, 101, 121
avocadoes 20, 24
awareness, field-based 111
awareness flow 108
axions 7
Ayurvedic approach 148–9

baking 66; during COVID pandemic 89
banking 80, 85
BBC Food Programme 129, 167
beans 20–1, 25, 28, 117

beliefs, core 68
Berger, John 61
Berne, Eric 41, 130
berries 24, 79
Bettelheim, Bruno 57
Big Ag 76
Biklé, Anne 77, 166
biotin 8
Black Lives Matter 96
blood-brain barrier 8
Blyton, Enid 144
borlotti beans 21, 28
Bourdain, Anthony 131
brain: and food 7–8; use of term 6
brain development 23, 43
bread 9, 21–2; wholemeal 101
breadcrumbs 88
breast feeding 31
breast milk 23, 55
Brexit 85, 129
British diet: and diverse cuisines 38, 93; traditional 20, 25, 37–8
broccoli 24
BSE (bovine spongiform encephalopathy) 81
Büber, Martin 64
Buddhism 40, 42, 62
bulimia 32–5, 38
burnout 141

caffeine 9, 19
calories 16, 24, 34, 68
Cambodia 97–8
Camilleri, Andrea 144
cancer 21, 32, 35
capital, distributed 126
capitalism 79, 83–5, 90, 100, 124–5
carbohydrates 18, 21–2; brain's use of 7; and metabolism 26; refined 59, 101, 121
care, unpaid 125

Carrara 132
Carrington, Damian 76
Carson, Rachel 81
cartesian theatre 39−40
catastrophizing 42, 74
cave paintings 11, 141, 151
cheese 22−3, 147
chefs 131; celebrity 12, 99, 116
chewing 55−6, 63, 65, 67−8, 154
chicken 20, 25
chickpeas 14, 21, 28, 117
chocolate 53−4
Christmas 12, 84, 152
cicoria 155−6
cities, evolution of 81−2
class 12, 100
climate change 93; and food production
    21, 23; food security and inequality 164;
    personal reflection on 91−2
colonialism 11, 97−8
the commons 126
communities: evolution of 79−80; meals
    uniting 152; wellbeing of 126
competence 104, 157; limits to 160
competence framework 12−13, 18
conflict 127, 157−60
connectedness 57; continuity of 60
consciousness: models of 106−9; shifts in
    105−6
contact, sphere of 133
contact boundary 57, 59−61, 74; in case
    studies 66−7; and consciousness 108−9;
    disturbances of 65; experience at 62;
    increasing awareness of 69−70; and
    societal change 114
cookery classes 28, 145
cooking: development of 79; outsourcing
    34, 99
Covid-19 pandemic 85, 88−90, 93; and
    food supply 11, 56; neighbourhood
    responses to 126; and on-line work
    133−4; social impact of 122−3
creativity 52, 108, 133; access to 143; and
    difference 159
cuisines, global variety of 24−6
cultural norms 93
culture, shared 12, 53, 129, 145
cytokines 9

da Vinci, Leonardo 110, 144
dairy products 20, 23
Damasio, Antonio 42
data, regulating intake of 122, 128, 138

David, Rachel 116
DDT 81
de Beauvoir, Simone 99, 144
death 35, 152−3; food after 143; and grief 46
deforestation 23, 77
dementia 101, 121
denial 10, 91, 121
Dennett, Daniel 39−40
depression: and diet 8, 36, 101, 121; and
    fats 23; and starvation 26; and stress 122
derivatives 85, 121
Descartes, René 39−40
desensitization 67
desire 54
despair 39, 42, 52, 91
diabetes: and Covid-19 89; type 2 35, 101
difference 11, 95−7, 99; and conflict
    158−9; fear of 105−6; and gender 99;
    social perception of 114
differentiation 63
digestion, water in 19
digital assistants 122, 130
digital trading 121
digital world 119
disabilities 100−1, 114
disruptors 159
diversity 108; integrating 95−6
Diwali 12
DNA 8, 26
domesticity 99
drama, and food 144
dualistic thinking 96−7
Dust Bowl 81−2

eating disorders 10, 31−4, 39; resources
    on 165
economics 122−5; capitalist 78−9, 83, 85,
    90; doughnut 125−7; and health 121
Eddo-Lodge, Reni 97
eggs 8, 23−4; boiled 149; protein in 20
ego, in Gestalt 55−6
ego states 41, 48
Egocentric attitude 107
Eisenhauer, Nico 77
Eleusis, Mysteries of 150
Embedded Economy 125
embeddedness 114−15
emotional, use of term 6
emotional injury 35−6
emotional range 43, 45, 74, 158
emotional satisfaction 53
emotions 42−3; case studies of 45−7; and
    the mind 43

empathy 6, 61, 133
environment 48; and consciousness 106,
    108–9; destruction of 79; and food
    production 18, 21; in Gestalt 50, 52–7,
    60, 62–4; interconnection with 3, 6, 9,
    11–12, 147; wider 18, 56, 69, 74
Epsom salts 24, 101
Equal Pay Act 98–9
equilibrium, disturbing 62–4
eros 147–8
essential services 89; accessing online 119,
    133–6
ethics 18, 80; codes of 119, 135
Ethnocentric attitude 107
European Association for Gestalt Therapy 105
excitement and growth 61
exercise 2, 101–2; lack of 36
experience: cycles of 64–5; elements of
    63–4; in Gestalt 60–2
expertise: of author 5; professional 135;
    technical 112

Facebook 116, 124, 159
FaceTime 89, 138
face-to-face interactions 122, 132–3,
    135–6, 138–9
families, conflict in 159
families of origin 21, 29, 43, 46–7
family festivals 152
family intervention 161
Farmer's Markets 139, 155
farming: origins of 80; *see also* agriculture
farming techniques 9–11, 77, 81, 101
'Fat is a Feminist Issue' (Orbach) 98
fats 18, 20, 22; and metabolism 26
fatty acids 20, 23–4, 101
Federman, Adam 132
fertilizers 3, 77, 81
feudal system 80
fibre 18–19
Field Theory 109–14, 126–7, 129, 137
figure and ground 61
finance, global 11
fish 7, 20–1; oily 20, 22, 24, 27, 101
Fisher, M. F. K. 153
flour 9, 80, 89
Floyd, George 96
folic acid 8
folk tales 149, 151
food: as art 145–6; and contact boundary
    59; digital 121, 129; feelings about 10;
    global trade of 85; impact on brain and
    gut 7–9; language of 3; and satisfaction

of needs 52–3, 74–6; social aspect
    of 28; still life paintings of 143, 153;
    thinking about 9–10
food avoidance 38
food choices 3, 5; unhealthy 29, 35–6
food culture 22, 27, 53
food environment 16–18, 26, 76
food groups 16, 18–24
food intake, regulating 16, 31–2
food porn 147–8
food production: economic and political
    structures of 76, 137; global 81;
    industrial 18; unsustainable 121,
    129–30; and water 87
food security 157, 160, 164
food shops, during COVID pandemic 89
food supply 56, 76, 82, 90
food writing 145
Freud, Sigmund 47, 54–5
fruit 7, 11; and the environment 19–20;
    importing 82; paintings of 143
futures 85

Ganesh 41
garlic 14–15, 38, 52, 72, 88, 117
Gates, Bill 129
gender 98–100; and class 100; and
    emotions 43; transcending binary of 107
gender identity 95, 102–3
genetic engineering 121
genome editing 129–30
Gentileschi, Artemisia 149
gestalt 50; ealry stages of formation 70;
    use of term 61
Gestalt psychotherapy 5, 50; eating
    metaphor in 55–7, 63, 65, 67–8; food
    in 65; historical background 54–5;
    language of 105, 108; non-dual thinking
    in 97
GI (glycaemic index) 7
gig economy 85
Gilligan, Carol 107
ginger 36, 117
global financial crisis of 2008 122–3
glucose, brain's use of 7–8
Goodman, Paul 54–5
grace 152
grains 7–8; and inflammation 9
gratitude 152, 163
greenhouse gas emissions 86
Grey, Patience 132
grief 43, 45–6, 150
grocers, ethical independent 127

gut: and food 8; use of term 6
gut microbiome 6, 8–9, 78, 101

Hammond, Liz 143, 161
health, models of 2
health professionals 12, 28–9; and anxiety
    about the future 124; and artificial
    intelligence 122, 130; and digital
    world 119; and genetic engineering
    121; limits to competence 157, 160;
    on-line interactions with 133–5, 138;
    supervision for 160–1
heart attacks 35
heart disease 101, 148
helping professions 5, 96
Hestia 149–50
Hodgson, Di 65
Holy Communion 150, 154
hospitality 106
households, in doughnut economics 125–6
Hughes, Mary 37
hummus 49, 117, 155
hunger 3, 16, 31; dying of 32; in Gestalt
    55–6; and satisfaction 53–4
hunter-gatherers 79, 99, 123, 141
hyperactivity 23

I-It 64
impairments 95
Indian cooking 93, 113
inequalities 83, 86, 89–90, 100, 157, 164
inflammation 9, 35–6, 101
information: diet of 128; factual 135;
    shared sources of 129
insomnia 24, 38
Instagram 14, 116–17, 144–5
integration 63, 107
intelligence 104, 128, 130; artificial 122,
    130–1
intention 54, 151
interconnectedness 31, 50, 53, 57
internal critic 44–5
internal process 41, 60
introjecting 65
intuition 52, 111
investing time and energy 53
irritable bowel syndrome 101, 116
Islamic faith 150
Italy 14, 22, 25, 104, 132
I-Thou 64

Jacka, Felice 8, 26
Jewish food 150

joints, swollen 35
just-in-time 83

Keats, John 146
kitchen, as sacred space 151–2
Klein, Naomi 164
knowledge: and information 128; and
    on-line work 133; types of 135
Korn, Leslie 18, 25–6, 35, 160

labour: and automation 131–3; and capital
    78, 83–5
land: as commodity 78–9; enclosure of
    83–4; ownership of 80–1
language 103–7; and metaphor 57; racist
    and sexist 114
'The Last Supper' (da Vinci) 144, 150
Lawrence, D. H. 144
Lawson, Nigella 99
leftovers 59, 88, 92
lentils 14, 20–1, 25
Lewin, Kurt 52, 109
Leyse-Wallace, Ruth 18
Liebig, Justus von 81
life spaces 109–11, 158–9
lifestyle diseases 10, 100–1
literature: and film 145; and food 144
Locke, John 80, 86

magnesium 24, 101
Manet, Edouard 146–7
Marchetti, Arianna 132
'the market' 85, 121, 125, 139
Marx, Karl 124
Mason, Paul 124
Mayer, Emeran 40
meals: shared 144, 152, 154; social media
    pictures of 145
mealtimes: preparing for 71; as rituals 151,
    163; and satisfaction of needs 53
meat 20; and art 11; cellular 129;
    industrialized production of 21;
    nutrients from 7–8
medicine, food as 148–9
meditation 42
Mediterranean diet 18, 25–6
Melchert, Norman 39
memories 27, 59, 111
mental health: conditions for 157–8, 162;
    maintaining 29, 126, 151;
    on-line resources for 139; and world
    crisis 93
metabolism 26

metaphor: of contact boundary 57, 59;
    food as 65
microorganisms 6, 8–9, 77–8, 166
milk: industrialised production of 23;
    transporting 82
mind, use of term 6
mindfulness 42, 163
minerals 18, 21, 23–4
Monalisa 62, 110
money 83; origins of 80
monkey mind 40
monosodium glutamate 155

National Food Strategy 10
nationalized industries 84–5
natural resources 11, 86, 121
needs: human 50, 52–4, 56, 137;
    meeting 65
negroni sbagliato 149, 156
neighbourhoods, conflict in 159–60
neoliberalism 79, 85, 124
Netflix 128, 159
neurodiversity 97, 101
neurons 6–7
neuroscience 5–6
neurotransmitters 7–8, 22, 24
newspapers 128–9
NHS (National Health Service) 32, 36, 85,
    88–9; website 9, 22, 24, 26, 33, 35
nitrogen 77
non-dual thinking 96–7
nourishment 3, 16, 26, 55, 74; and
    capitalism 79, 123; emotional and
    psychological 33, 147; from information
    121–2, 128; of otherness 158
'now,' current experience of 60
the numinous 53, 146, 151, 153
nutrition: and fats 18, 22; and food groups
    16; and mental health 27–8; and nuts 24
nutritional types 16, 26
nuts 8, 21–2, 24, 38

oats 49
olive oil 14, 72; importing 82; in
    Mediterranean diet 25, 38
Oliver, Jamie 99
omega-3 fatty acids 20, 24, 101
onions 14, 72; red 117
on-line meetings 132
on-line psychotherapy 138–9
on-line work 122, 133, 137
Orbach, Susie 98
organizations, structure of 112

Ostrom, Elinor 126
otherness 99, 158
Ottolenghi, Yotam 117
overeating 32, 34, 163
overweight 10, 32, 34–5; and COVID-19
    89; and disability 101

Packham, Chris 101
palm oil 23, 88
pan-scrapers 49
Parkinson's disease 8
Parks, Tim 6
Parlett, Malcolm 109–10
Passover 150
pasta 21–2, 25, 38, 89
peas 20–1, 163
perfectionism 45–6
Perls, Fritz and Laura 54–6
permeability 66, 108
personal reflections 14, 27–8, 37–8, 48,
    70, 91, 116, 138, 154–5, 162–3
pesticides 3, 77, 81, 123
philoxenia 106
plastic 23, 72, 88, 91–2
Poli, Piergiulio 48
politics: and economics 79, 123–4; and
    food 11
pollution 19, 113; and autism 101;
    economics of 127; and food production
    21; and inflammation 35; and soil 77
pornography 147–8
porridge 8, 18, 25, 37, 49, 149
post-traumatic stress disorder 36
potatoes 7, 20–2, 25, 101, 163
poverty 34, 90, 145, 155
privileges 23, 96–7, 99–100, 103–5, 108
probiotics 9
processed food 9, 27, 34; and cancer 35
Procyk, Anne 35
proflection 66
proteins 7, 9, 18, 20–1; and metabolism
    26; vegetable and animal 21
psychological, use of term 6
public spaces 84
pulses 15, 20–1, 25

Quantum Theory 54, 109

race 12, 95–7
Ramadan 12, 150
Rashford, Marcus 89
Ratcliffe, Rebecca 97
Raworth, Kate 125–7, 132–3

red kidney beans 21, 28
reflective practice 13–14, 137
Reich, Wilhelm 55
relational environment 41
relational field 50, 110
relational styles 39, 56–7
relationship with food 2, 6, 29–32;
    addressing 39–48; family's 161;
    personal reflections on 13–14, 70–1;
    resources on 165; societal 10, 76, 79–83,
    88–90; in therapy 66–8; unhealthy 27,
    33–9; and with the world 122
relationships with others 16, 18
religion, and food 149–51
resilience: building 2, 74; and crisis 93;
    and family of origin 29
resource list 165–8
restaurants 56, 99, 113, 131, 146
rice 21–2, 25; brown 7, 22, 101
ritual meals 53
rituals 2; secular 12, 53, 145, 151
robots 122, 131–3
Roden, Claudia 150
Roman Catholic Church 12, 150, 154
Rovelli, Carlo 54
Russell, Ken 144
Ryde, Judy 96

saffron 36
salmonella 81
salt 3, 22, 25; superstitions of 149
schizophrenia 8, 23, 36
school dinners 37–8, 83, 89, 123
seasonal foods 25
self: bodily 67–8; and environment 57;
    sense of 39; use of term 7
self-harming 39
self-isolation 39
self-talk 42
sell-by dates 87
senses: and food 11; use of term 7
serotonin 7–8, 76
sex, and food 146–8
sexual behaviour, unsafe 39
sexuality 93, 95, 102, 114, 119
Shah, Jo 127
shame 10, 39, 91; dying of 32
shellfish 20
shopping, and voting 139
Sicily 20, 25, 107, 155
Sikhs 150
Siri 122, 130
Skype 89, 124, 138

Slater, Nigel 99
slavery 96, 150
sleep: disturbed 26, 42; and inflammation
    36; and neurotransmitters 7–8
Smith, Adam 125
social media 10–11, 115–17, 137–8;
    overload from 122; sharing information
    on 128–9, 145
societal change 93, 112–15
soil, nutrients from 9–10, 76–8
sourdough 3, 9, 117
Soviet Union 124
spirituality, and food 12, 141
spitting out 38, 56–7, 63, 65, 67–8, 128
starvation 26, 88
Steel, Carolyn 79–84, 165–6
Stein, Gertrude 102–3, 144
Stein, Rick 146
street parties 152
stress 122; coping mechanisms for 19,
    38; and inflammation 36; and lifestyle
    diseases 101
stress response 9
stroke 35, 101
stroke theory (TA) 130–1
Stuart, Tristram 87
sucking 55, 63
sugar: and colonialism 97–8; refined 7, 9,
    100–1
supermarkets 76; supplying 82–3
superstition 149
swallowing 63, 65, 67–9
synapses 7

taste, categories of 155–6
teeth 55–6; and calcium 24
Thatcher, Margaret 85
thinness, extreme 32, 34
thirst 19
thoughts 29, 31, 39–42
Thunberg, Greta 101
Toklas, Alice B. 102–3, 144
Tomasi, Carla 14
tomatoes 25, 36, 155; tinned 72, 89
tone, emotional 112
trade unions 84–5
trans fats 101–2, 121
Transactional Analysis 41, 48, 130
transcendence 53, 74, 151
transport infrastructure 11
transportation of foods 82–3
Trump, Donald 85, 105
turmeric 36

umami 37, 155
United States, farming techniques of 81
us and them 105–6
Usher, Sharon 154

value: monetary 85–6, 121; nutritional 88,
  128; redefining 100
vegetable fats 22, 101
vegetable protein 21
vegetables: and art 11; avoiding waste
  of 87–8; and the brain 7–8; and the
  environment 19–20; importing 82; and
  soil nutrients 10
verbal cues 136
virtual realms 130
visual art 143–4, 146–7
vitamin B6 8, 24
vitamin B12 24
vitamins 8, 18, 21, 23–4

Wabi Sabi 143
walnuts 8, 24, 49
waste 86–8; at the dinner table 37, 59

water 18–19; and food production 86–7
Wheeler, Gordon 105–6, 166
whole foods 14–15, 27
wholemeal flours 22
Wikipedia 6, 126
Wilber, Ken 107–8
wine 12, 18; importing 82; in Mediterranean
  diet 25; microbes making 77
wisdom 128, 149
Wood, Amanda 162
work environments 103, 111, 115, 159
work fields 112
working from home 125–6, 136; *see also*
  on-line work
Worldcentric attitude 107, 114
Wrangham, Richard 79

yoga 40, 42, 148
yoghurt 9, 23, 49, 113
YouTube 40, 106, 126

zinc 8
Zoom 89, 132, 138, 144–5

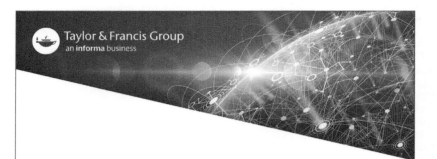